Challenging the Indian Medical Heritage

CEE **Environment & Development Series**

Sustainable Development in Fragile Environments, *N.S. Jodha*

Sustainable Technology: Making the Sardar Sarovar Project Viable, *Suhas Paranjape* and *K.J. Joy*

Waste Minimization: A Practical Guide to a Cleaner Production and Enhanced Profitability, *Prasad Modak*

Joint Forest Management: The Haryana Experience, *Madhu Sarin*

Banking on Biomass: A New Strategy for Sustainable Prosperity Based on Renewable Energy and Dispersed Industrialization, *K.R. Datye*

Minding our Marine Wealth: An Appraisal of Gujarat's Coastal Resources, *N.D. Chhaya*

Nurturing Biodiversity: An Indian Agenda, *Madhav Gadgil* and *P.R. Seshagiri Rao*

Renewable Energy and Environment: A Policy Analysis for India, *N.H. Ravindranath, K. Usha Rao, B. Natarajan* and *P. Monga*

Towards an Agroecosystem Policy for India: Lessons from Two Case studies, *A. Damodaran*

Water Harvesting and Sustainable Supply in India, *R.N.Athavale*

Challenging the Indian Medical Heritage

Edited by

Darshan Shankar and P.M. Unnikrishnan

Foundation for Revitalisation of Local Health Traditions
Bangalore

Centre for Environment Education

Ahmedabad

FOUNDATION BOOKS

Delhi • Bangalore • Mumbai • Kolkata • Chennai • Hyderabad

Published by
Foundation Books
4764/2A, 23 Ansari Road, Daryaganj, **New Delhi** - 110 002

FOUNDATION BOOKS
C-22, C-Block, Brigade M.M., K. R. Road, Jayanagar, **Bangalore - 560 082**
Plot No. 80 Service Industries, Shirvane, Sector-1, Nerul, **Navi Mumbai - 400 706**
60, Dr. Sundari Mohan Avenue, 1st Floor, **Kolkata - 700 014**
21/1 (New No. 49), 1st Floor, Model School Road, Thousand Lights,
Chennai - 600 006
House No. 3-5-874/6,4, (Near Apollo Hospital), Hyderguda, **Hyderabad - 500 029**

The **Environment and Development Book Series Project** is funded by the Swiss Agency for Development and Cooperation and managed by the Centre for Environment Education (CEE). CEE is a national institute, established in 1984, and supported by the Government of India, Ministry of Environment and Forests.

Project Committee	:	Kartikeya V. Sarabhai, Seema Bhatt, Kiran Desai, Prithi Nambiar, Bipin Shah
Project Coordinator	:	Prithi Nambiar
Project Team	:	Maitri Baruah, Snehalatha S.V, Snehal Bhatt
Editorial Assistance	:	Sarita Vellani
Layout	:	Balamani R. Menon
Photographs	:	Brand E advertising
Cover Design	:	BRAND EQUITY

Jointly published by Foundation Books and the Centre for Environment Education.

ISBN 81-7596-187-2

Published by Manas Saikia for Foundation Books and Printed at Print Perfect, Mayapuri, New Delhi.

Foreword

The Centre for Environment Education is concerned with bringing more innovative strategy to the notice of policymakers and the general public in order to sensitize them to the need for environmentally sound decisions. The current book series has been planned as a means of providing access to alternative viewpoints, backed by analysis and information on various policy aspects presented by development theorists and practitioners from diverse fields.

There is considerable rhetoric about the value of knowledge available in our traditional systems but this is yet to translate into a practical attempt to make this knowledge viable and usable in the present context. The country's indigenous medical traditions include both the codified system of Ayurveda, and folk tradition, which is passed from one generation to another orally. Both systems yield knowledge on prevention, cure and health promotion. Ayurveda in Sanskrit means *"the Science of Life"*. It is an ancient system of treatment based on medicines prepared from herbal plants found in abundance in India. Ancient knowledge systems of medicine provide the basis for alternative preventive, curative and restorative treatments that have gained increasing global acceptance. These knowledge systems seek to maintain the balance of the physiological systems in a holistic way to prevent diseases and revitalize the body, mind and soul.

The book discusses some of the indigenous traditions of Ayurveda and folk medicine that are of practical value and calls for the revitalization of medical traditions through careful documentation, testing and collection of evidence that supports epistemological as well as contemporary user value. The author is of the opinion that while little effort has been made to evaluate or introduce rigour in the testing of these indigenous systems, formal education continues to favour western "modern" knowledge over tradition.

The author reviews traditional practices that could contribute to new developments in medicine and examines possibilities for collaborative research between modern medicine and traditional medicine. There is much to be said for "medical pluralism" which is becoming a reality in today's world. But as the author points out, the contemporary relevance of traditional medicine lies in its potential to supplement and strengthen the maintenance of health in a broader and decentralized way. At the policy and practical level, there is much that needs to be done to enhance the range of medical options available and to strengthen delivery systems through education, scientific rigour and demonstration.

Kartikeya V. Sarabhai
Director
Centre for Environment Education

Foreword

I first became involved in exploring local health traditions in India as part of my work on immunisations as advisor to Rajiv Gandhi in the late 1980s. At the time, we were researching and investigating alternative forms of medicine and their potential for immunising India's masses against disease.

It was in this context that I first met Darshan Shankar, who embodied a wealth of knowledge regarding India's rich medical history and traditions. Together, we set up the Foundation for the Revitalisation of Local Health Traditions, with the goal of reviving alternative and traditional medical practices as a way of providing health care. The Foundation promotes the concept of Indian self-reliance in primary health care, and opens the door for unique contributions from India to the larger medical world. My involvement in the Foundation has been extensive and is an ongoing learning experience.

Traditional medicine has vast potential in today's technologically advanced and fast-paced society. In the most advanced nations, the general public no longer believes that any 'single' medical system can solve all their health needs. There is a growing acceptance that medical pluralism, based on 'best health practices and theory', holds the key to the future of health care. This trend is reflected in the rapid growth of what is termed in the West as the 'Complementary and Alternative Health Movement'. A focus on Indian medical science would demonstrate confidence in our expertise, and assert our independence in charting out a unique course for medical discovery that is all our own.

India is distinctively positioned to create this vision for effective, pluralistic health care, based on our rich indigenous medical heritage and traditions. This book is authored by knowledgeable and committed individuals, who have been working diligently towards the revitalisation of our medical heritage. They are both insightful and visionary in their outlook, and write with clarity and passion, demonstrating their commitment to establish a unique contribution by India to global medical practice. As the book shows, local health cultures represent a high degree of decentralisation in peoples' medical care — one that aids millions of rural and urban homes in becoming self-reliant. The task of reviving India's long-dormant medical heritage and realising its overwhelming benefits is a large yet important one — and efforts like this represent a first and effective step at meeting that challenge.

Enjoy.

Sam Pitroda
10-12-2002

Acknowledgements

Several competent colleagues, reputed NGOs and village communities of Karnataka, Kerala, Tamil Nadu and Maharashtra have contributed to the writing of this book. Chapter 4 on 'Building a Bridge Between Local Health Cultures and Codified Traditions' has been written by A. V. Balasubramaniam, Director, Centre for Indian Knowledge Systems, Chennai, while Balasubramaniam and Ram Manohar have provided inputs for the chapter on 'Alternative Macro Visions'. Chapters 6 and 7 have been largely written by A. Hafeel and T.S. Suma of the Department of Traditional Systems of Medicine, FRLHT. We also wish to acknowledge the technical inputs and timely help rendered by Asmita Wele, Roohizaman, Rajalakshmi and Vijayakumar for the chapter 'The Materia Medica of Ayurveda'.

'Health at Our Doorstep' (Chapter 8) has been contributed by G. Raju and G. Hariramamurthy, with inputs from Anthodaya Sangha (ANSA), Covenant Centre for Development (CCD), Gandeepam, Social Change and Development (SCAD), People's Agricultural Farm (PAF), League for Education and Development (LEAD), The Peoples' Federation, village resource persons (VRPs), *natti vaidyas* (NVs), Siddha doctors, schoolteachers, kitchen herbal garden (KHG) growers, Anantanarayana Sarma, Lakshmi Rahmathullah and her associates from Aravind Hospital for Women, Children and Community Health, Madurai.

Chapter 9 ('Our Living Medical Heritage') has been written by various colleagues: 'Trisivaperur's Poison Specialist' has been written by A. Hafeel; 'Mantrada Thirumalaiah' by B.S. Somashekhar; 'Ankola's Miracle Workers' by Joel Deepak D'Silva; 'Nativaidya Narayana Murthy' by R. Prabha; 'Ten Generations of Eye Physicians' by M.B.Gayatri, M. Abdul Kareem and Sarbeswar Kar; 'The *Pasu Vaidya* of Kadari' by M. Abdul Kareem, Harish Bhat and Prabhakar Achar; and 'Traditional Bonesetting' by Vishnu Mathur and Meera Rammohan.

For one whole year, T.S. Suma and A. Hafeel invested a lot of time and energy coordinating with the authors to come up with the initial draft of the manuscript. We would also like to express our gratitude to Sugandhi Rani J,

Vidya Venkatesh, Mangala, C.K.N. Menon and Hema Padmini for painstakingly keying in the manuscript sent by the authors.

The idea of writing this book came up during the Documentation and Rapid Assessment Project (DALHT) supported by ETC-COMPAS of the Netherlands, which has also given the FRLHT team financial support for both writing and editing this book. We thank Bertus Haverkort, Wim Hiemstra, Katrein Van't Hooft and Coen Reijnties of the COMPAS team for their encouragement and inputs.

We deeply appreciate the extremely insightful editing and critical suggestions offered by Manoj Nadkarni and Nikhil Govind. The prologue and epilogue would not have been written but for Manoj's insistence. The insightful editorial inputs for the chapter on 'Community-based Oral Health Traditions in Rural India' by Nikhil have added to its quality. We would also like to thank Madhav Karki, who reviewed the manuscript and whose critical comments we incorporated into the book.

Even after a long spell of editing, the manuscript had a number of loose ends. These were identified and rectified during the final editing by Ms. Sarita Vellani. Her inputs have been extremely vital for the book. We thank her immensely for the same.

Finally we would like to place on record our heartfelt thanks to Sam G. Pitroda, who has written the Foreword.

Darshan Shankar
P. M. Unnikrishnan

Contents

List of Tables

List of Figures

List of Boxes

SECTION I
Perspectives on Indian Medical Heritage

Prologue

Darshan Shankar

As an urbanite, I had studied the natural sciences in school, college and university. However, these were all of Western origin: I was not exposed to any other form of knowledge. I did not know that other useful knowledge systems — indigenous ones — existed in an organised form in our society or that they were still functional and used regularly by a vast number of people.

Later, while working as a social activist, I lived in the Karjat tribal block for 12 years. There, for the first time, I encountered medicinal plants and forests. I could not fail to notice, often with amazement, that the local *Thakur, Mahadev Koli*, and the *Katkari* tribals used many local plants and animals for health care. The methods of treatment I saw first-hand were incredible and impressed me deeply. Lactating mothers used *Ipomoea mauritania (vidari kand)* to enhance breast milk. The leaf of the common plant *Calotropis gigantea (arka patra)* was used to reduce a testicle swollen to twice its size (presumably hydrocele): the treatment worked in four days! The latex of the same plant applied on the skin could draw out a thorn from deep within. The fruits of *Terminalia bellirica (bibhitaka)* were used to treat dry cough. The roots and bark of *Holarrhena pubescens (kutaja)* could cure dysentery. *Helicteres isora* (*muradasinge* in Marathi) could stop diarrhoea. The 'touch-me-not' plant *(Mimosa pudica* or *lajjavanti)* was used to stop uterine bleeding, and the juice of *durva* grass (*Cynodon dactylon*) could dissolve gall bladder stones.

I discovered that the tribals of this area knew the uses of over 400 plants, animals, birds and reptiles. The people who had access to and used this kind of knowledge were ordinary householders as well as more specialised village healers. Often, households knew of home remedies for managing more than 30 common health conditions. Every village had a birth attendant (called *sueen*) and at least one other socially recognised healer whom the villagers called *vaidu* (healer). There were *vaidus* who specialised in treating snakebites, others specialised in treating broken bones, and there were those who treated veterinary problems. None of the *vaidus* depended on healing for their livelihood. They had other occupations and healing was only a social service.

Once, when a colleague of mine was suffering from a severe bout of jaundice, I consulted a *vaidu*. He promised to get me a remedy the next day. In fact he did not show up for two days. He then cheerfully explained that he had to go deep into the neighbouring forests to locate the herbs he needed. He had spent two whole days looking for the plant, which was used by my colleague with dramatic results. The healer, however, did not ask to be compensated for the trouble he had taken. It was left to us to express our satisfaction in whatever way we could afford. In the tribal culture, no patient expects 'free service' and they show their gratitude by giving the healer some grain, a hen, or a bottle of the local brew; but all this is not demanded as a precondition for the service.

I asked university-based phytochemists and pharmacologists their opinion of these practices and if they could scientifically verify these remedies. They had no clinical data on the applications of these materials. In few cases, the chemistry of a plant was known and the biological activity of an active compound had been studied on rabbits or mice. This information was not sufficient to validate tribal practices. The tribals did not just use active compounds — they used flowers, fruits, bark, root, latex and gum, either in combination or in their entirety. Chemists and pharmacologists unfortunately did not know anything of the biological activity of the entire plant, only of certain chemicals derived from it. The scientists I approached worked in reputed institutions. However, they could not help. They needed huge funds and several years of research to carry out systematic studies. Hence in my pursuit of validation for local health practices, I was led to the traditional physicians of Ayurveda (the word itself means 'Science of Life').

The Ayurvedic physicians I met impressed me. They knew the materials the tribals had used and had books on indigenous pharmacology *(Dravya Guna Sastra)* in which the materials had been studied using 10 to 15 different parameters. They could therefore confirm the validity of tribal treatments. At times, they could suggest modifications to the local practice, or even substitute plants in cases where the original plant was not available. These doctors knew the systemic effect of plants, their metabolic effects at different stages of ingestion, and their action on body tissues, organs, etc. They also knew the side effects and contraindications as well as how to cancel them by adding other natural substances to balance, synergise or improve their assimilation. I was surprised by the depth of their knowledge, which included processes required to convert plants into various dosage forms and strengths.

I was deeply impressed by the attitude and conduct of an eminent Ayurvedic physician from Pune. He was publicly felicitated for curing a case of leukaemia: the patient, who had been given a few weeks to live, had survived without remission for five years and was still healthy. While speaking at the felicitation, the physician declared:

> "Ayurveda does not have a term equivalent to 'cancer' and there is no mention of a condition called leukaemia. I did not bother to study the case sheets and the diagnosis from the cancer hospital that my patient presented to me for scrutiny because I have not studied biochemistry and therefore do not understand the subject. I examined the patient afresh and diagnosed his condition using Ayurvedic principles. The patient's status had to be classified under a provisional diagnosis that was not described in the diagnostic literature of Ayurveda (Ayurvedic science does enable physicians to make provisional diagnoses of new health conditions that have not been previously described). I then designed a treatment to suit my diagnosis. The patient was thus cured."

He added:

> "I do not, however, claim to be able to cure cancer. But I do claim that I have the capacity and willingness to look at any new health condition for, with the help of Ayurvedic science, a physician may be able to diagnose and treat, and perhaps even cure the disease."

This statement gave me an insight into the dynamic nature of Ayurvedic science.

Using the context of pharmaceuticals, I observed that although the manufacturing technology behind indigenous medicine was pre-industrial, the logic behind dosage forms like wines, *bhasma*s (baked powders) and oils was sophisticated. The number of traditional methods of processing was far more than those available in other medical system. I appreciated the range of the diagnostic acumen of traditional healers — their reading of the pulse, for instance, appeared incredibly sophisticated. Their acute clinical observations, even for a simple condition like a cough, were impressive. According to them, a dry cough was a wind disorder, a cough with heavy congestion and expectoration was due to an imbalance of water and earth, and a cough with inflammation and sore throat and mild congestion was due to an imbalance of *agni* or fire. These are all expressions of a scheme of 'systemic' diagnosis. In this scheme it is not important to identify a causative agent like a virus or bacteria, which may in fact be present, but to read from the symptoms the specific nature of systemic imbalance that has taken place and to choose for treatment natural products that will restore the balance. Scientists may subsequently discover that this scheme of treatment might also inhibit the growth of bacteria and virus in unexpected ways.

As an Indian citizen, my exposure to the rich culture and knowledge of my own people both inspired as well as angered me. I felt inspired by the decentralised nature of folk health knowledge. Rural India already appeared to have the futuristic ideal of 'health in your own hands' that social thinkers dream of. Every village household had the knowledge of dozens of common ailments and also of preventive and promotive health care aimed at introducing practices that result in total health rather than only in fighting individual illnesses. Along with this, every village has its own folk healers who have the appropriate skills to manage most primary health problems.

It is extremely important to note that folk traditions are not only rooted in the community, they are also supported by the community. The size of the folk tradition in any locality, and thus all over India, is so large that it is only the whole community that has the capacity to sustain the tradition. In the 1980s the Health Ministry made the mistake of declaring that they would pay Traditional Birth Attendants (TBAs) for every delivery conducted. It soon found out that state governments could not afford to pay thousands of TBAs. Nor was it easy for them to monitor such a process. So today, the estimated 600, 000-plus TBAs of India continue to be paid by their own communities.

I also felt proud to see that, apart from the folk tradition, there was another stratum to the Indian medical heritage. This comprised the codified traditions, which are based on sophisticated theoretical foundations. These codified traditions appeared to have a symbiotic relationship with the folk tradition.

From the Karjat experience, I could infer that Indian medical traditions have an amazingly large resource base. In the Karjat tribal block itself, which covers an area of 30 sq km in a dry, deciduous forest, the tribals had knowledge of the medicinal uses of around 400 plants and a dozen birds and animals.

But along with this pride, I also felt anger that this wisdom and these traditions were being neglected. The younger generation in Karjat was not keen to be apprenticed to healers, and respect for the *vaidu* tradition outside the tribal setting was quite low. Even in the institutionalised tradition I observed that the level of self-confidence and self-esteem of *vaidyas*, *hakims* and *siddhars*[1] is quite low. This is because educated Indians do not regard them as highly as they deserve. I asked myself why mainstream students and teachers in schools and universities do not engage in studying indigenous knowledge when it is so rich and relevant; or why outstanding physicians of the folk or codified systems are not sufficiently respected and honoured in their society. I was saddened by the fact that ethnic communities are not encouraged to continue with their amazing innovations.

These feelings kindled in me a desire to do something to revitalise Indian medical traditions and demonstrate their contemporary relevance. Thus, the years since 1984 have been spent in trying to work at the grassroots as well as regional and national levels in the pursuit of this dream. In 1993, with the help of a very open-minded telecommunications engineer, who is also a great nationalist, I established the Foundation for the Revitalisation of Local Health Traditions (FRLHT). Over the last eight years, FRLHT has done some pioneering work in conserving the plant resource base of Indian medicine. It has also built up valuable databases on the traditional codified knowledge of plants and initiated pilot projects — like the kitchen herbal garden programme — in peninsular India for revitalising folk medicine.

[1] Doctors in other systems of medicine are called by these titles.

This book is a response to those initial feelings of pride and anger. It is an attempt to introduce to the lay reader the medical traditions that exist in India. This is done along two lines. The first is to provide the reader with a general introduction to the codified (or classical) systems of medicine, including their recent history and their theoretical foundations. For this, one system — Ayurveda — is examined in some detail. The second addresses the neglect of these medical traditions, calling for urgent action to counteract this. The latter part of the book describes the work being done to document and revitalise the folk medical tradition. Brief sketches of some outstanding folk practitioners are also included.

Apart from myself, the authors who contributed to this book are practising Ayurvedic doctors and researchers working in the field of traditional medicine. We hope that the present work will serve its purpose and make clear the need for conserving and enriching traditional systems of medicine in India. If we ignore their value and their wisdom, it will be as great a loss to the world as to India.

There is a wealth of knowledge in both the folk as well as codified stream of traditional Indian systems of medicine — knowledge that deals with prevention, health promotion and cures, giving each dimension equal emphasis and providing practical advice regarding all three aspects. The folk stream knows of the medical uses of over 8,000 species of plants, as well as of several hundred species of animals, minerals and metals. It is estimated that there are around 40,000 herbal and natural product formulations known and used in the folk tradition. This stream is a treasure trove of nutritional information about thousands of ecosystem-specific food resources that are documented in modern books on the subject. It also has a unique knowledge of the therapeutic and processing techniques of local resources.

The extent of knowledge possessed by the codified stream is reflected in the large number of medical manuscripts and the range of subjects they cover. Physicians, scholars and seers have generated an ocean of classical medical knowledge. This is in addition to the information drawn from the empirical knowledge of the folk stream. Apart from knowledge of drugs, there is extensive knowledge of diagnostic methods, therapeutic techniques, surgery, specialised lines of treatment, physiological concepts, as well as an understanding of the body–mind relationship. There are an estimated 50,000 herbal formulations in the traditional formularies of Ayurveda alone. Unfortunately, there is no comprehensive catalogue of Indian medical manuscripts. They lie scattered in Oriental libraries and in private custody — not only in India but also in Sri Lanka, Nepal, Burma, Mongolia, China and Thailand, as well as in the libraries of Western Europe and the USA. This situation is indicative of the severity of neglect of the Indian medical heritage by both our state and central governments. Other potential patrons, too, seem indifferent.

It is estimated that there are over one million medical and non-medical manuscripts in all Indian languages in collections all over the world.[2] However, there is no estimate regarding the number of manuscripts in the area of medicine. The Tamil University in Tanjore carried out a preliminary analysis of all Tamil manuscripts in public collections in India and other parts of the world, and their work shows that there are a total of 24,000 extant Tamil manuscripts. Of these, 4,000 are on medicine. In this context, we must bear in mind that these are in addition to the substantial number of manuscripts that exist outside of public collections, in the families of practitioners.

Traditional Indian systems of medicine have their own theoretical foundations, worldviews, methods, logic, principles, concepts and categories, which are quite distinct from Western knowledge systems. That these systems were alive and well until the beginning of the twentieth century is borne out by the nineteenth century Ayurvedic studies recorded in *Nighantus*[3] of the properties of exotic plants like tea, coffee, green chillies, brinjal, tomato, potato, pineapple, etc., which entered Indian soil only in the last 200 years.

The existence of large amounts of readily usable reference materials might lead one to assume that their importance is well recognised. Unfortunately, this is not true. Both the folk medical culture and the codified classical health

---

[2] Personal communication with Kapila Vatsayan, Director, INTACH, New Delhi.

[3] *Nighantus* are lexicons. Those published in the eighteenth century document the properties of exotic plants like green chillies, potato and tomato on 'Ayurvedic' parameters, thus indicating that the science was creative during this period (after which, and particularly in the twentieth century, there has been a 'lull' in terms of new applications).

systems are being eroded. This erosion is especially alarming because it does not appear to be on account of medical inefficiency; it has more to do with economic, cultural and political factors. In part, it is due to the suicidal attitude of the Indian elite and policymakers, who ignore and even discourage serious research on the theoretical foundations of indigenous medicine. Ironically, such work is well under way in many Western universities.

These are other telltale 'signs' that point to the erosion. In the folk tradition the erosion is evident at the household level in the reduced use of home remedies, traditional diets and health customs. There is the classic example of the plant *Phyllanthus amarus*,[4] which is called *keezhanelli* in Tamil and *bhumi amalaki* in Sanskrit. While traditionally, this plant was widely used for jaundice (*kamala*) by rural households all over southern India and the Andaman and Nicobar Islands, today it is used by very few rural folk. This is certainly not because the plant is medically ineffective. Recently, an American Nobel Prize winner claimed a patent on the use of the aqueous extract of the whole plant as a safe drug for Hepatitis B&C. This brings home the point that the erosion of folk health traditions has more to do with cultural and sociological processes rather than 'medical efficacy'. We need to either strengthen the tradition or destroy it if it is useless. But we simply cannot afford to ignore it.

The erosion of folk traditions is also evident in the age profile of contemporary folk practitioners. In all the categories of folk practitioners — TBAs, bonesetters, herbal healers, veterinary doctors and the like — the average age is above 40. This is indicative of the declining interest in folk traditions over the last two decades.[5]

Compared to the last century, there does not seem to be any significant drop in the number of physicians (487,000)[6] in codified practice. However, the levels of self-confidence of the practitioners, as well as the quality of

---

[4] US patent No: 4, 673, 575; date of patent: 16 June 1987; composition, pharmaceutical preparation and method for treating viral hepatitis – Ventkateswaram.P.S., Irving Millman, Baruch.S.Blumberg, Assignee – Foxchase Cancer Centre, Philadelphia

[5] Based on data from micro-studies. *Tribal Traditions of Karjat Tribal Block* (2000) edited by R. M. Nanal and published by the Academy of Development Science, Maharashtra.

[6] This is the figure of ISM physicians given in the latest draft of the National Policy on Indian Systems of Medicine published by Ministry of Health, Government of India in 2001.

their knowledge, seem to have declined significantly. This assessment, although subjective, has been consistently reiterated by leaders of the codified tradition in various internal reviews through the last century right up to the present time.

What are the causes of this erosion? The folk medical system has depended almost entirely on community and family support. Its erosion does suggest some degree of loss of confidence of the community in its health traditions, which has impacted the morale of the practitioners. Random social surveys have revealed a certain prejudice among the younger generation regarding the efficacy of traditional knowledge as against the supposed reliability of modern knowledge. This prejudice has perhaps been inadvertently nurtured by the formal education system in schools and universities. But alongside the erosion, there still remain some who are faithful: else the tradition would have completely died out.

Actually, there has been no systematic effort to evaluate the codified medical knowledge. Nor has any appropriate cross-cultural research methodology been developed for assessing indigenous knowledge. Ignorant commentators declare the codified medical knowledge systems to be unscientific and consider this to be a crippling deficiency. In terms of epistemology, Indian Knowledge Systems are different and unlike Western science, and in that sense may perhaps be labelled unscientific. The Western scientific knowledge system, however, is only one cultural way of knowing nature. There are also other cultural ways of knowing nature that are equally effective, and the codified Indian medical knowledge systems illustrate one such alternative. Since there also has been no serious and balanced attempt to defend indigenous medical knowledge, this epistemologically uninformed prejudice continues to prevail. Practitioners and scholars of the codified traditional medicine systems, who could be expected to defend themselves, are too demoralised to do so.

Meanwhile, in the last 200 years, the scientific, economic and political influence of Western biomedicine has been overwhelming and has affected all sections of society, including the tribals. They have also been strongly influenced by advertisements. They are deeply impressed by neatly packaged pills and syrups, and the magical injections that efficiently anaesthetise. The 'government' doctor, who only practices Western biomedicine, wearing an impressive white coat with a stethoscope around his neck, and who also often expresses his disbelief in '*jadi buti*' (herbal stuff), reinforces this attitude.

While the application of Western medicine has provided relief for several problems and great strides have been made in surgery, the prejudice against indigenous medicine has led to some glaring distortions in the faith of the public in its own traditions. There was a time a few years back when rural mothers were led to believe that powdered milk was superior to breast milk; or that the neatly packed and expensive electral formulation was superior in controlling diarrhoea than the traditionally used soup of boiled rice and lentils; or that a bottled soft drink is a better option to offer a guest than tender coconut water; or that storing drinking water in copper vessels purifies the water is just a blind belief. However, studies by Padma Venkat and her colleagues at the FRLHT Laboratory show, beyond a shadow of doubt, that micro-organisms like ecoli, fungi and algae present in water get completely destroyed within six hours of storage in copper vessels and that the level of copper that dissolves in the water is far below what WHO prescribes as toxic.

The loss of self-confidence of practitioners in the codified tradition, too, has been partly due to reduced social support and partly due to the totally irrational demand that they 'justify' their knowledge by Western biomedicine parameters. If the situation were reversed and Western doctors were asked to prove the efficacy of their practice on the indigenous knowledge parameters of *panch maha bhutas*,[7] one can well imagine their plight. While it is unfair to expect the average physician of one medical discipline to be proficient in another, intercultural work needs to be encouraged at least in specialised centres. In this case, the paradox has also been compounded because of insufficient state and private patronage for foundational or intercultural research work on Ayurveda. This has resulted in sub-critical investment during the last 100 years in formal education, research, manufacturing and health services. Indian systems of medicine even today receive less than 3 per cent allocation of the national health budget.[8]

[7] The five basic states of matter referred to in Indian systems of medicine.

[8] See Seventh, Eighth and Ninth Five Year Plans for Indian systems of medicine, approved by the Planning Commission, Government of India.

The erosion of indigenous medical knowledge has taken place not only in India but also in other countries around the world. The reason in all cases is attributable to cultural, economic and political processes, but not medical inefficiency. At a global level, the World Health Organisation (WHO) spends less than 0.1 per cent of its worldwide health budget on indigenous medical systems.[9]

If we accept the view that indigenous medical knowledge is not facing erosion on account of its insufficiency or incapacity, we must admit that given its vast knowledge base, it has tremendous potential to contribute to health care. A strategy for the revitalisation of Indian medical heritage must be thus urgently promoted.

The 'mantra' for a revitalisation strategy should be medical pluralism. One core premise behind this idea is that any single medical system is bound to have its limitations and, therefore, the best health solutions that different systems can offer in supplementary and complementary ways should be used. The health needs of people the world over will be best served if every country encourages a policy of medical pluralism. This means that our strategy should not pit indigenous knowledge against scientific knowledge, or traditional medicine against Western biomedicine. Rather, it should promote plurality and the integration of medical systems at every level of health services. There is, in fact, a growing public demand for such integration all over the world, which has been responsible for the dramatic growth of the movement for complementary and alternative medicine.

But can collaboration with Western biomedicine help the Indian medical heritage? The short answer is that it could help explain the value of the Indian medical heritage to the Western world. It could stimulate indigenous practitioners and shake them out of their inertia. It could provide novel solutions to difficult health problems that have incomplete or no solutions in other systems of medicine. However, it would be impractical, unaffordable and wholly unnecessary to attempt to translate all traditional knowledge into Western science. Such an exercise would be unnecessarily time consuming and the cost would be immense — it takes US$ 200,000 and 8 to 10 years to validate a single new

---

9 Personal communication with Professor Gerard Bodekar, Chairman, GIFTS, Oxford.

drug. Furthermore, the 'translation' would be imperfect and incomplete because of the basic incompatibility of paradigms.

There is reason to believe that traditional physicians have some outstanding practices that can contribute to expanding the frontiers of medicine. For example, traditional bonesetters in India can straighten a clubfoot without surgery. They also make use of bamboo and wood splints for flexible bandaging of a fractured limb. Leading orthopaedic surgeons are now suggesting that the Plaster of Paris casts have several limitations while the use of splints or flexible bandaging offers a definite advantage. Indian bonesetters are experts in this field. A WHO report states that in China they have been able to significantly reduce the time taken for recovery from bone fracture by using a combination of modern and traditional bone setting practices.[10] The traditional knowledge of *acupressure* (*varmam* in Siddha and *marma* in Ayurveda), *nadi pariksa* (the science of pulse diagnosis) and specialised therapeutic areas like *panca karma* and *rasayana* are other examples of subjects that can help to make original contributions to the world of medicine.

However, whereas collaboration with Western science might help explain some aspects of traditional medical knowledge to the Western world, it cannot revitalise indigenous medical knowledge or help Indian medicine recover its creativity. That will be possible only when the indigenous knowledge system becomes self-generating again.

For over a century, collaboration between traditional medicine and Western science has been on a very unequal footing. Generally, most efforts have concentrated on picking up bits and pieces of information from traditional medicine and incorporating them into a Western framework. This has not led to a wholesome growth, or even strengthening, of traditional medicine, nor has it provided Western biomedicine with balanced solutions. For example, take the case of the plant *sarpagandhi*.

The roots of the plant *sarpagandhi* (*Rauvlfia serpentina)* are used by traditional medicine in an admixture of several compounds for certain conditions

---

[10] *Traditional Medicine & Health Care Coverage* by E. D. Robert and H. Bannermen (1983). Geneva: World Health Organisation.

such as mental disorders. The discovery of the traditional drug was based on indigenous pharmacological science (called *dravya guna shastra*). About 100 years ago, modern pharmacological investigations were started on this plant, which culminated in the isolation of an alkaloid that was named *Reserpine*. It was trumpeted as a scientifically proven product and marketed for several years as an improvement over the traditional use.

However, scientists soon found that the so-called pure drug *Reserpine* has a number of side effects, which are not experienced when the patients used the whole aqueous extract of *Rauvlfia serpentina* root powder.[11] Moreover, the industrial production of *Reserpine*, obtained by purifying the *Rauvlfia serpentina* plant, also made great demands on the supply of the plant. The result was that the wild population of this plant declined and it is now on the list of endangered species. The environmental cost of large-scale manufacture of herbal medicines is only now beginning to be recognised as a serious limitation to herbal drug development.

While integration at the level of health 'services' does suggest collaborative research, it certainly does not mean a merging of different medical knowledge systems. It means exploring functional bridges for communication, ethical collaboration and mutually beneficial cooperation across medical systems without any interference with their autonomy. Collaboration between medical systems can make the best progress when the parent medical disciplines are also active and flourishing in their own right.

Today, apart from Western biomedicine, the use of all other medical knowledge systems is only marginally encouraged; this bias needs to be urgently corrected. This is essential; for it is mainly due to lack of political support that non-Western knowledge systems have so far failed to establish their 'right' to development. Their methods and methodologies lie

[11] One is likely to face similar problems with the use of 'piperine', a purified compound isolated from the plant *Piper longum*, which the Council for Scientific and Industrial Research (CSIR), Government of India, has recently patented for its ability to enhance bio-availability of certain synthetic drugs. This work is based on the lead derived from Ayurveda about the *agni*-enhancing action of the plant, but scientists have not bothered to go into the contraindications associated with the prolonged use of *Piper longum*, which are also pointed out in the Ayurvedic materia medica.

unexplored outside of their traditional worlds and their universal applications are ignored. It is alarming to see that they are, in fact, being further marginalised due to the renewed political and economic effects of globalisation that, in its current form, has its intellectual and philosophical roots in mainstream Western cultures.

It must also be pointed out that, although not flourishing, indigenous knowledge continues to be alive, and hence evolving, changing and adapting. Only dead things do not evolve and change. The concern for the revitalisation of indigenous culture must thus be viewed not as a concern for blindly reviving the past, but rather as a serious attempt to broaden and deepen the scope, quality and content of modern civilisation. Unfortunately, over the last two centuries, the process of modernisation has got wedged into a narrow monoculture track based almost exclusively on the Western cultural and intellectual tradition. Monoculture is dangerous for the survival and evolution of civilisation. Uniformity narrows down the alternatives and options available to the peoples of the world, as well as their capacity to cope with the present or prepare for the future.

All countries have a potential stake in supporting the revitalisation of indigenous cultures because the world civilisation as a whole stands to gain from a state of flourishing cultural diversity. The key to appreciating cultural plurality is an acceptance of the fact that cultures are guided by their own way of looking at the world and acquiring knowledge from it. It seems to be necessary to appreciate the historical fact that various knowledge systems have had their genesis and basic evolution in specific cultural spaces in time and hence are bound to be different in their expression.

Modern science, as we know it today, is in this context definitely a product of European culture. Modern Western medicine, therefore, cannot be viewed as the only valid form of health care. To understand this, we shall first need to study, even if briefly, the epistemological, political and cultural background of traditional systems of medicine. We shall do this in two different forms; the systematic codified form of Ayurveda and the non-codified one of folk traditions. We hope that our understanding of Ayurveda can, for the most part, be extrapolated to the other indigenous knowledge systems of the world, at least to make the point that knowledge rooted in different cultures may function and perform on the basis of different worldviews and that so long as that knowledge is seen to deliver useful advice, products and services to humankind, it is worthy of policy support, even if its 'expressions' and experiences are very different from the expressions of Western science.

1

Community-based Oral Health Traditions in Rural India

Darshan Shankar

Any attempt to introduce local health traditions is handicapped from the start due to their oral nature and the seeming absence of a theoretical foundation. It would seem that the test of their efficacy lies only in empirical evidence. In other words, for the most part they are merely considered to be a somewhat more sophisticated version of the trial-and-error method based on keen local observations. It is observed that many village healers do not care to generalise about how or why their method works. This is seen as evidence that the local traditions lack the theoretical rigour of either Ayurveda or modern medicine.

One way of addressing the issue — and this is part of the approach of this book — would be to assert that the local traditions are empirical manifestations of the underlying theoretical structure of the classical tradition itself. There is no doubt that village healers often use procedures, the elaborate explanations of which are located in chapters and verses of Ayurvedic texts. This gives us an immediate sense of the marvellous interpenetration of the classical and village traditions —villagers perhaps know that theoretical explanations are frequently justifications of what they are doing. It has been repeatedly found that, having observed procedures being performed by a village healer, researchers work backwards merely to find their elaborations located in the classical tradition. On the other hand, it often seems that without the visible and expert performance of the village healer, the classical tradition seems only a maze of complex theory and obscure formulae. By observing the village healer, one identifies possible wedges that might enable one to prise open the wisdom of ancient generations.

Nevertheless, it may be appropriate to insert a word of caution here. The exact modalities of the continuity between the classical and the vernacular traditions are very far from being fully established. Much mutual borrowing and enrichment has no doubt taken place. Yet any pronouncement on the precise nature of their relationship is still far away in the future and requires much more detailed scholarship.

In India this issue is, of course, part of the larger question of the relationship between the classical and the vernacular. For our purposes it is relevant only insofar as it relates to local health practices. A later chapter gives examples of how local practices of diet can be understood in terms of an Ayurvedic rationale. But even in this limited context, it is important that such investigation be pursued, even if the practitioners (at the level of the household or of the village physician) are unaware of the rationale that underlies their practice. It is equally important that such investigations are not rendered so rigid or narrow as to preclude the possibility that these practices might have been derived from an unrelated epistemology. What is vital is not so much to explain the emanation of the village system from the classical system (or vice versa), but to fulfil our need for medical pluralism; in short, to keep open all doors so that the greatest possible variety of reliable choices are available to the consumer of health services. Just as Allopathy must not be allowed to 'squeeze out' the native tradition, so, too, must Ayurveda and the other written traditions not be allowed to pre-empt the possibility that some local traditions may be of independent and autonomous origin. We feel it necessary to make this disclaimer before we begin our tentative explorations.

The Need for a Basis

For any kind of exploration of local traditions, it is important to take into account the disappointing state of research on folk medicine under the larger rubric of medical research. To begin with, non-codified traditions are hardly treated as medical traditions. But initial attempts at foundational research into the classical systems have been equally disappointing. Here, the issue is clearly one of failure of our public health policy. Given the size and spread of folk tradition, a thorough investigation of its roots and practices is essential in the public interest. This orientation in policy and research can be possible only if medical institutes offer courses related to the living traditions, including their philosophical origins. What needs to be studied are not merely practices but also, if only at a preliminary level, issues related to a cosmo-vision of folk medicine — for example, the spirit in nature, the orientations of the self in space and the triangular grid of mind–nature–body. We can no longer afford to see such issues as academic. Without the local and the codified indigenous streams relating at this level to Allopathic assumptions, we simply cannot hope for any progress in the field of medical pluralism. Philosophy is not merely a convenience that can be discarded at will to attend to the putatively more 'practical' aspects. Theory is integral to every level of practice.

We hope, therefore, that in the future, serious research on folk medicine will become a priority of any institute devoted to the advancement of Indian medicine. For this, a 'foundational' approach that will enable a fresh understanding of both the classical and folk systems is the only approach that will be equal to the task. The uncovering of the epistemology of the folk is more difficult than the recovery of the classical. Even today, many aboriginal healers do not know (or care) why a certain plant heals a certain disease. In such cases it is up to the medical researcher to attempt a discovery of underlying patterns. This would require not only patience but also vigilance, for it is necessary to resist the temptation to make large generalisations that yield only short-term gains. A full investigation into the ecology of health practices must attempt to find all the links and interrelationships of such practices; in other words, their observation might require going beyond the question of health per se, to related questions of lifestyle, diet and cultural practices in general. In the process, the question of health might well lead to an exploration of a new way of 'living out' the relationship of the mind–body–nature triangle. In principle, at least, such issues ought not be considered entirely outside the purview of an investigation into the creative springs of the folk tradition. Health in all its ramifications — inner, outer, sociological and cultural — must form an integral part of the syllabi of institutes of medicine.

Discovering Oral Health Traditions

As we know, community-based, oral health traditions are embedded in the lifestyle, diet and health practices of thousands of local communities all over India. Like music and agriculture, health care also flourishes as a folk tradition. It is estimated that there are around 1.4 million folk healers as well as millions of rural (and to a much lesser extent, urban) households who possess immense knowledge of home remedies. They are also well informed about local foods, their availability and nutritional value. The health traditions of all these healers are based on local resources. According to an All India Ethno-biological Survey carried out by the Ministry of Environment and Forests, Government of India, over the period 1985-1995, around 8,000 species of wild plants were listed as being used in health care by rural and tribal communities. These account for almost 50 per cent of the known flowering plants of India (17,5000 species). Apart from plants, local animals, metals and minerals are also used.

The most fascinating features of local health traditions are their wireless (non-institutional) transmission and the fact that they are self-sustaining. They exist in millions of homes and thousands of villages, town and cities, without the aid of any institution or external source of funding. They are transmitted through family or community traditions via a person-to-person process. Folk *gurus* (teachers) guide their *sisyas* (students) in cultural and ethical codes, which evolve, adapt and alter in time. They embody the knowledge of the human mind, physiology and anatomy as well as of food and nutrition. This knowledge extends even to the pharmacological properties of plants, animals, metal and minerals. Though community health practitioners have no legal status, they enjoy much social legitimacy in their localities.

It must be noted that folk healers do not generally undertake medical service as a full-time vocation, nor are they dependent on their health services for a livelihood. The typical healer may be a farmer, a barber, a shopkeeper, a blacksmith or even a wandering monk. And while the medical services they provide are not free of charge, they are offered in an ethical and non-commercial spirit. So though the community (patient) pays the healer for his/her services following local cultural norms, the income earned is usually incidental and supplementary. This low sustenance cost is one reason why the tradition is so large, widespread and decentralised, and has over million foot soldiers. If folk healers were to depend on such earnings for their livelihood, their numbers would have been much smaller, as not every village can sustain the livelihood needs of full-time healers.

The health traditions of a community must also be distinguished from their other health practices. A community may have several current health practices, such as the use of aspirin for headaches, but these do not fall under the ambit of tradition. Traditions comprise practices that are self-perpetuating and transmitted without the intervention of any agency or institution. They are often passed down orally or in a written form through generations of the same family or community.

An example of a seventeenth century health diet tradition of northern India is the dish made of potatoes (*Solanum tuberosum*; Hindi name: *aloo*) and *methi* (botanical name: *Trigonella foenum-graecum)*. This dish is prepared by thousands of households and is referred to as *methi–aloo* (and not as *aloo–methi*). This is to stress the use of a higher proportion of *methi* to *aloo* on the logic that *methi*, by virtue of its 'hot' nature, balances the wind-producing effect of the potatoes. This example also points to the dynamic and adaptive nature of local health traditions. Potatoes are not native to India and were introduced into the country by the Portuguese in the sixteenth century. The material was studied and assessed by Ayurvedic physicians who found it to be 'wind' producing and advised that it be eaten in combination with other balancing materials like *methi, jira* (*Cuminum cyminum)* and *hing (Ferula asafoetida).*

Another example of an ancient health food tradition that is still alive and flourishing is the highly nutritious South Indian '*idli*', a steamed cake made up of rice and lentils. The lentil used in *idli* is *masa (Vigna mungo)*, which, though rich in protein (*mamsa vardhaka*), is also hot and acidic (*usna* and *pitta karaka*). In North India, it is only eaten in winter; were it to be eaten in summer, it would cause hyperacidity and flatulence. The South Indians, however, have overcome this problem by cleverly combining *masa* with rice in a certain proportion (1:3). The dish is then prepared using the fermented dough of these two materials.

Having thus eliminated the side effects of *masa*, the *idli* can be eaten throughout the year. With a healthy balance of protein, carbohydrates and vitamins, it is easy to digest and can be eaten by the old, young and even infants. The *idli* is an ideal health food, the preparation of which is part of a living tradition known and practised by millions. In India, one can find a tremendous range of such regional diets. While the various ethnic communities use only ecosystem-specific food resources, these are far more numerous than those documented by food and nutrition textbooks.

Apart from the oral traditions at the household level, there are widespread health traditions that are practised on a community scale. Every village in India has a few traditional birth attendants (TBAs) or midwives. These midwives can handle breach deliveries, laterally positioned foetuses and infants with their umbilical cord displaced around the neck. They can even deliver a stillborn child. India has around 600,000 such TBAs who are maintained in villages through apprenticeships that extend from generation to generation.

Amazingly, India also has a folk orthopaedic tradition. Every cluster of 20–25 villages has a bonesetter. These bonesetters treat sprains and simple fractures, and in some parts of the country they also manage compound fractures with open wounds. There is no systematic study available on them yet, but it is obvious from the low access to hospitals available in rural India that traditional bonesetters manage most broken bones in the villages.

Local health practitioners do not just deal with general health problems. There are also community traditions relating to emergencies — as is evident from the existence of an estimated 60,000 healers who treat poisonous and even life-threatening snakebites.[12] The traditional *visa* (poison) healers can distinguish a poisonous snakebite from a non-poisonous one and, further, between the bite of a krait, pit-scaled viper, Russell's viper and a cobra, each of which merits a different treatment. In some regions they also treat those bitten by mad dogs to prevent rabies.

Finally, there are about 100,000[13] herbal healers who treat a range of common ailments, chronic conditions and even specialised conditions related to the eyes, ears, skin and muscular and nervous disorders.

All these are 'health traditions' because they survived, evolved and adapted themselves over centuries. There is no single medical school or agency that is responsible for the transmission of this knowledge, either at the household level or at the level of the specialised folk healer; it has spread through personal contacts.

---

[12] Extrapolation from micro-studies carried out by Foundation for Revitalisation of Local Health Traditions (FRLHT), Academy of Development Sciences (ADS), Lok Svasthya Parampara Samvardhan Samithi (LSPSS)

[13] Extrapolation from micro-studies carried out by Foundation for Revitalisation of Local Health Traditions (FRLHT), Bangalore, Academy of Development Sciences (ADS), Karjat, and Lok Svasthya Parampara Samarthan Samithi (LSPSS), Coimbatore.

However, there has been serious erosion in many segments of this tradition. Having become aware of this, it is necessary to develop an operational strategy that will revitalise the informal educational process as well as the community support system that has upheld the tradition for centuries. In this context it is very important to understand that any intervention that intends to strengthen community health practices must also protect their autonomy and self-reliance. It is only the local communities of India that can support both their own health traditions as well as their local transmitters. Local and central governments and Non-governmental Organisations (NGOs) can provide local communities support, but they should take care to do so without hobbling or crippling the tradition itself.

How is this to be done? India's oral health traditions are vast, covering thousands of natural resources, plants, animals, minerals, wild vegetables and fruits. They encompass several preventive, promotive and curative health practices. It will easily take more than a century to fully document and assess the numerous and diverse health practices in every corner of the country. Yet, if these traditions are to be revitalised, it is important to prioritise certain health practices and initiate their assessment in order to generate confidence in the community regarding their value. For this, it would be essential to design an assessment methodology that is sensitive to, and takes into account, the basis of local knowledge systems. We cannot impose evaluation schemes based on paradigms that are incompatible with local epistemologies. Furthermore, different approaches may be needed for traditions related to (*a*) food and nutrition, (*b*) health customs, (*c*) preventive and promotive practices, and (*d*) curative health practices.

Historically, oral traditions have had a symbiotic relationship with the codified Indian systems of medicine (ISM) like *Ayurveda, Siddha, Unani* and *gso-rig-pa*. If these oral traditions are to be revitalised, it may be useful to restore and promote their functional relationship with these ISM. This would need a carefully worked-out strategy based on the realisation that while it would be disastrous to suffocate the oral traditions with the theoretical burden of formal medical systems, Indian medical systems as well as modern medical science could, if creatively applied, contribute to the revitalisation of our oral health traditions.

There is one other problem that would need to be addressed: the 'ownership' of traditional health knowledge. While it appears to be minor blip at the moment, it may become more threatening in the future. In countries outside India most problems relating to traditional knowledge and biopiracy pertain to oral health traditions. These traditions do contain valuable experiences that are vulnerable to exploitation by medical research and commerce. There is, thus, a need to spread awareness regarding the property rights of the traditional custodians of health knowledge, but in a balanced way, without creating paranoia. Model Material Transfer Agreements (MTAs) and Information Transfer Agreements (ITAs) would have to be evolved to protect the intellectual property rights of community knowledge. But this would have to be done based on the realisation that benefits from the commercialisation of a few amongst the thousands of available local health practices that are indeed commercially viable, is not going to make rural communities wealthy. The real benefits lie in the active use of these practices for self-reliance in primary health care. The need of the hour is therefore to create an environment that would foster local innovations based on local knowledge systems.

2

Alternative Macro Visions

Darshan Shankar, P. Ram Manohar and P.M. Unnikrishnan

It is unfortunate but true that international cooperation in 'science', defined in its broadest sense as approaches to a systematic study of nature, does not exist across different world cultures. Whether Chinese, Indian, African, South American or Western, scientists today are all members of the same scientific club. And while scientific institutions have been established in different geocultural regions, their work is completely insulated from their own indigenous sciences, which may be based on very different ways of knowing nature.

We begin by citing a striking example of the fallacious conclusions that can be arrived at in cross-cultural studies. In his monumental work, *Science in Traditional China,*[14] no less an authority than Joseph Needham concludes that while the technological contribution of the Chinese to the world has been diverse and impressive, its 'shortcoming' lies in that it did not culminate in 'science'. The ethnocentric assumption of Needham is that Western scientific expression is the preferred and highest mode of flowering of any knowledge system. There are similar conclusions by European scholars regarding the nature and status of Indian contributions to mathematics, medicine and astronomy.[15]

While the worldviews of the Indian folk as well as codified medical traditions overlap, they are both very different from the worldview of Western medicine. This difference is not surprising as the genesis of Indian medicine, both in terms of time as well as the cultural space in which it evolved, is so different from that of Western medicine. To understand this fully, we would first need to understand the theoretical basis of the Indian medical heritage and appreciate its cultural underpinnings.

---

[14] *Science in Traditional China—A Comparative Perspective* by Joseph Needham (1981). Hong Kong: Chivere University.

[15] A good discussion of these issues can be found in *Indian Science and Technology in the Eighteenth Century* by Dharmapal (1971). Hyderabad: Academy of Gandhian Studies

The Indian tradition comprises such medical knowledge systems as *Ayurveda, Siddha, Swa-Rigpa* (Tibetan) and *Unani*, as well as folk systems. These (except for the folk) are all codified systems with sophisticated theoretical foundations and a special understanding of physiology, pathogenesis, pharmacology and pharmaceuticals. The contents of Ayurveda, for instance, cover eight broad areas: *Kaya cikitsa* (general medicine), *Bala cikitsa* (paediatrics), *Grha cikitsa* (psychiatry), *Urdhvanga cikitsa* (ear, nose, throat and eye), *Salya cikitsa* (surgery), *Damstra cikitsa* (toxicology), *Jara cikitsa* (rejuvenation) and *Vajikarana cikitsa* (virilification).

In indigenous pharmacology, better known as *Dravya guna sastra,* the entire plant and/or its parts — the leaves, stem, seeds, root, bark, fruit, flowers — are studied as a whole in terms of their *in vivo* 'systemic' effects on such parameters as *rasa* (taste, of which there are six, each suggestive of the composition, properties and biological activity of the substance), *virya* (the potency of a substance immediately after ingestion), *vipaka* (the post-digestion state of a substance) and *prabhava* (the overriding biological activity of a substance), and used as therapeutic agents. Modern pharmacology, on the other hand, isolates an active chemical entity from the plant or its parts and studies its *in vitro* and *in vivo* effects on micro organisms or body tissues. Both approaches undoubtedly have their uses. The difference lies primarily in the fact that, in indigenous knowledge systems the evaluation is 'systemic', whereas in Western medicine it is 'atomic' or cellular; furthermore, the category of knowledge known as chemistry is absent and is substituted by another category called *Dravya guna sastra*.

In any comparative study of the two sciences it is imperative to have an appropriate terminology and language for a dialogue. Correlations between the medical systems are, however, poorly established at present. For instance, *vata* is often equated with the nervous system or nerve force, and *pitta* with the digestive system, enzymes, hormones and the heat-regulating mechanism. While such an equation may work at one level, it often breaks down at other levels. The intellect, for example, is a function of *pitta,* representing a preponderance of *satva guna* (a term that refers to a quality of the mind). In Western physiology, however, the intellect falls in the domain of the nervous system and must therefore be equated with *vata*. Such equations tend to be untenable because the principles of classification in Western medicine and Ayurveda belong to radically different orders. When Western physiology speaks of nervous tissue, muscular tissue or epithelial tissue, the principles of classification are anatomical, based on the structure of the component parts. In the Ayurvedic triadic classification of *vata, pitta and kapha*, the basis is biological and based on systemic functions.

To cite another example of incompatibility, the essence of the modern laboratory method is to first isolate an object or aspect from its environment, eliminate temporarily its links with other diverse factors in nature, and then reduce its relationships to engage the minimum possible number of measurable and controllable parameters. These parameters are then varied (usually one at a time) and their effects on the object studied. Finally, there is an attempt made to integrate the findings arising out of the disintegrated studies.

In contrast, the traditional approach attempts to solve a problem by considering it in its entirety, including its interlinks and outside connections. This method of solving problems in their natural setting seems to be efficient in providing balanced solutions. Indian systems seek to study nature by systematising natural phenomenon and to make it rigorous rather than destroy its essential unity and multifaceted character. Thus, according to *Caraka*, Ayurvedic science is dependent upon *yukti*, which is the method that perceives phenomena brought into existence by the coming together of a multiplicity of causes. Having perceived this multiplicity of causes, it uses *yukti* to bring about holistic understanding and design appropriate actions and material at the appropriate time and place. Thus, the traditional system, even in its theoretical formulation, seeks to find a holistic strategy for healthy living rather than dissecting life and then trying to string it together again. It appears, then, that while traditional sciences are built upon a stupendous amount of detailed and minute observations, they do not have a disintegrated scheme for experiment in the modern laboratory sense of the term.

To elaborate further on the differences in approach: the Ayurvedic analysis of matter is in terms of *panchabhutas*, that is, the five sense impressions resulting from the contact of matter with the sense organs (sound [ear] attribute of space; touch [skin], attribute of air; form [eye], attributes of fire; taste [tongue], attributes of water; smell [nose], attributes of particulate matter, i.e., earth). The Western method, on the other hand, analyses matter according to the chemical elements of which it is composed, and is therefore objective. From a philosophical standpoint, the subjective analysis provides the advantage and satisfaction of having a complete theory valid for all time because sense functions do not change (the attribute of *sanatana*).

Although measurement and quantification are an important part of indigenous systems of medicine, they differ in form from their modern counterparts. Most measurements in the traditional sciences are made using units 'normalised' to an individual. In *Yoga cintamani*, for instance, a *matra* of time has been defined as the time taken by a sleeping individual to complete one cycle of breath: one inhalation and one exhalation. Although measurement and quantification have their place in Indian Systems of Medicine (ISM), their role is different from that of modern systems. In India, it is not the geometry of Euclid but the *Astadhyayi* of *Panini* that is considered the supreme example of the construction of theory. Indian sciences are based on the understanding that numbers and symbols are not essential to achieve scientific rigour. Rather, the technical use of natural language –– Sanskrit, for instance — has sufficed, even in highly abstract and technical topics like logic, mathematics and *Vedanta*.

The Worldview

The Ayurvedic tradition views the world in terms of varying configurations of the 'five states of matter' present in all objects. These five states are viewed in a descending order and are symbolised by the words *akasa* (space), *vayu* (wind), *agni* (fire), *ap* (water) and *prthvi* (earth). All natural objects, living and non-living, consist of these fives states, albeit in different proportions. And just as the atomic configuration of a material determines its form and properties, it is these proportions that determine the form and qualities of every object.

These five states of matter are associated with the five human sense organs. It is the ear that perceives *akasa* through 'sound' vibrations that are its principal attribute. It is the skin that senses movement, which is the attribute of wind; the eyes that see and sense light — the attribute of *agni;* the tongue that tastes, which is the attribute of liquids (*rasa*); and it is the nose that smells as *gandha*, which is the principal attribute of solids.

In both the folk and codified traditions, properties of materials are expressed in terms of the material state dominant in them. Thus, the potato is wind or *vayu* causing because it is *guru* or heavy to digest and hence vitiates the wind. Chillies, on the other hand, have a higher proportion of *agni* or fire as the dominant state; the thinner the chilly, the spicier it is likely to be as fire in a fat chilly is balanced by its content of water. Again, the cucumber has relatively more water (or *ap*) as its dominant state and can thus boast of cooling properties.

Diseases are also seen as an imbalance *(vikrti)* in the normal proportions of the five states in the human body. Parkinson's disease or paralysis, where limbs tremble or become frozen, is due to an imbalance of wind *(vayu)* in the body, which affects motion. Hyperacidity is caused by an imbalance of fire (*agni*) and wind *(vayu);* obesity represents an imbalance of solid and liquid *(prthvi* and *ap*) states.

This indigenous worldview also believes in the existence of a subtle world of spirits *(bhuta, preta)*. The objects in this spirit world are known to be dominant in the space and wind principle *(tattva)*. The human mind — as opposed to the brain — is itself the manifestation of 'spirit' in the human body. The mind is *akasa* (space) and *vayu* (wind) dominant *(pradhana)*. Therefore, according to Ayurvedic theory, if the mind is to be influenced, it can be influenced by regulating breathing *(vayu)* or by using 'sound' in the form of music, *mantras* and thoughts. It can also be influenced by drugs that act on *akasa* (space) or *vayu* states.

In the specific context of Ayurveda and modern medicine, the difficulty in making comparisons becomes evident when one attempts to compare their internal parameters. For instance, there is no conceptual correlation available between the three basic physiological parameters of Ayurveda (*kapha, vata and pitta*) and the parameters of modern physiology, such as hormones, blood pressure, lipid levels, blood sugar and bilirubin levels.

Ayurveda also does not give quantitative parameters the same importance they receive in the Western tradition; although measurement and quantification are used, they differ in form from the Western systems of knowledge.

Most measurements in traditional medical science are made using units that are normalised to the individual. That is, while assessing a person's height or length of his or her limbs, the measurement is expressed in units of *anguli*, the dimension of a finger of the concerned individual. There is thus no arbitrary standard external to the individual, such as the international metre. Such normalised units exist not only for measurement of length but also for volume and time.

Again, while Ayurveda, like the Western systems, does have methods of verification, sophisticated schemes for diagnosis, descriptions of the evolution of diseases, as well as criteria for admitting a therapeutic substance into the materia medica, all of them are based on its own epistemology, which is different from that of the modern sciences.

The worldview of Ayurveda is based on the *sankhya* school. *Sankhya* assumes that the manifest or objective world (*vyakta*) emerges from the unmanifest (*avyakta*) or subjective world and that there is an essential unity and continuum between the two. At a philosophical level, it implies the essential unity of the inner and outer self and of nature. Thus, from the Ayurvedic standpoint, the realistic way to understand nature is by becoming 'one' with it.

We can do this by using our mental apparatus and the five senses that serve as instruments of knowing in a balanced way. The senses naturally move outwards to see, hear, touch, smell and taste. The mind can move both outwards with the senses or move inwards and experience an inner, non-sensory world. In the Ayurvedic literature there is reference to the *apta* or *seer* of the *sastra*, whose mind is both objective and subjective. A mind that is in control of the senses and is totally free of the six divisive prejudices[16] is said to be both perfectly objective and subjective. This is the mental state of *Brahma*, from which the Ayurvedic *sastra* was originally propounded. In such a state there is oneness with nature.

[16] According to the *Caraka Samhita*, the six prejudices are lust (*kama*), anger (*krodha*), greed (*lobha*), intoxication (*mada*), delusion (*moha*) and jealousy (*matsarya*).

At this point, it would help to demystify this mental state by pointing out that one can free the mind of the six prejudices through mental training of the sort described in the *yoga sastras* and in such texts as the *Patanjali yoga sutras*. In the Western tradition, too, mental training is essential for a seeker of knowledge. However, there is little systematic understanding of the different mental states; the 'scientific temper', which is meant to describe the ideal mental state of a scientist, is explained in general terms and scientific training is limited to the use of analytical disciplines like mathematics and logic.

The science of Ayurveda is based on the recognition of six fundamental *padarthas* or existential principles. These are *Dravya* (categories of being, of nine types), *Guna* (qualities, of 41 types), *Karma* (actions, of five types), *Samanya* (generic principle), *Visesa* (differential principle) and *Samavaya* (inseparability principle).

In the Western tradition, three basic existential entities are considered, namely, matter, time and space. In the Indian scheme of understanding, consciousness and mind are also existential entities. The expression of the manifest world is understood to evolve from the subtlest non-material state of consciousness (*atma*) to the grossest material state of *prthvi* (solid). Material and non-material existence is seen on a continuum.

Thus consciousness devolves into mind, and because of qualities like numerability (*sankhya*), magnitude (*parimana*), uniqueness (*prthaktva*), conjunction (*samyoga*), disjunction (*vibhaga*), nearness (*paratva*) remoteness (*aparatva*), impression (*samskara*) and casual relation (*yukti*), leads to the notion of time (*kala*) and space (*dik*) on the mental plane. The mind further devolves into the five states of matter, i.e., *akasa*, *vayu*, *agni*, *ap* and *prthvi*. All manifestations — small or big, subtle or gross, micro or macro, internal or external, organic or inorganic, living or non-living, unmodified or modified — are created by a permutation and combination of these basic categories and reflect the combined effect of their inherent qualities and actions, similarities, distinctiveness and inseparability.

The purely subjective mind is expected to lead to accurate perception and cognition of the subtler aspects of nature, whereas in the objective mode of knowing, the five senses and the rigour of logic (to process sense data) are used for perceiving the gross world. It is the combination of the subjective and objective ways of knowing that leads to a holistic understanding of nature.

Table 2.1

Tools of Knowledge and Their Applications (as explained in Ayurvedic literature)

Tools of Knowledge	Level of Application
Aptopadesa (Knowledge through teachings of seers who are one with nature)	*Tattva* (principle) and *Vyavahara* (practice)
Anumana (Knowledge through inference including *Yukti*–causal relations, and *Upamaan*–comparative reasoning)	*Sastra* (codification of knowledge)
Pratyaksa (Knowledge through direct perception including *yogaja pratyaksa* or intuitive cognition	*Vyavahara* (practice) and *Tattva* (principles)

Another distinction between the Western and Ayurvedic traditions is that while the former only considers direct perception, induction and deduction as the means of knowledge, a*ptopadesa* (knowledge gained by seers through revelation) is a distinctive feature of the Indian tradition.

The Ayurvedic definition of *svasthya* or health provides a good illustration of the holistic nature of the knowledge system. According to Ayurveda, the etymology of *svasthya* is to be established in oneself. *Svasytha* further implies equilibrium of body tissues, physiological functions, excretory processes, the senses and the mind. There is also the availability of sophisticated schemes that have been developed by Ayurvedic *sastrakaras* for diagnosis, clinical examinations and for the admission of drugs into its materia medica. The scheme for diagnosis includes an in-built early warning system. The different stages of a disease's development are recognised in the Indian tradition and its advancement can be checked when/if diagnosed by its prodromal indicators.

Table 2.2

Holistic Scheme for Understanding the Genesis of Diseases

Fivefold scheme for diagnosis	**Relation to stages of disease development**	**Illustration in the case of *amlapitta* - hyperacidity**
Nidana (aetiology)	*Caya* (accumulative phase)*Prakopa* (aggravation and activation phase)	*Viruddhanna* (incompatible food), *amlaseva* (sour food), *vidahyanna* (heat generating food), *pitta prakopakanna* (food that increases *pitta*)
Purvarupa (prodromal indicators)	*Prasara* (dissemination and repercussion phase) *Sthanasamsraya* (localization phase)	*Trt* (thirst), *daha* (burning sensation), *amlodgara* (sour reaction), *sveda* (sweating)
Rupa (full blown symptoms)	*Vyakti* (manifestation phase) *Bheda* (disruption and complications phase)	*Avipaka* (indigestion), *klama* (lethargy), *utklesa* (nausea) *tiktamlodgara* (bitter and sour eructation), *gaurava* (heaviness), *hrddaha* (burning in the heart), *kanthadaha* (burning in the throat), *aruci* (loss of appetite), *atisara* (loose bowels), *vamana* (vomiting), *moha* (delirium), *murccha* (loss of consciousness), *jathara vrana* (ulceration)

(contd.)

(Table 2.2 contd.)

Fivefold scheme for diagnosis	**Relation to stages of disease development**	**Illustration in the case of *amlapitta* - hyperacidity**
Upasaya (therapeutic response of diagnostic value)	Confirmatory tests	*Aharopasaya* Confirming diagnosis through responses to diet, medicine and behaviour
Samprapti (overall analysis of the manifestation of disease, understanding which helps to design treatment)	*Caya*, *Prakopa*, *Prasara*, *Sthanasamsraya*, *Vyakti*, *Bheda*	

A systematic diagnosis of a patient is expected to take into consideration a multiplicity of factors. These range from the status of the patient's various physiological states to inferences drawn based on the natural habitat in which the patient resides, his constitution (*prakrti*), mental state, and dietary habits.

Table 2.3
The Holistic Scheme of Diagnosis

Dosa (function)	*Vata*, *Pitta*, *Kapha*
Dusya (structure)	*Rasa* (plasma), *Rakta* (blood), *Mamsa* (muscular tissue) *Medas* (adipose tissue), *Asthi* (bone tissue), *Majja* (marrow), *Sukra* (reproductive tissue)
Desa (habitat)	*Anupa* (wetland), *Jangala* (arid land), *Sadharana* (moderate land)

(contd.)

(Table 2.3 contd.)

Bala (strength)	*Sahaja* (natural), *Kalakrta* (seasonal), *Yuktikrta* (induced)
Kala (time)	*Ksanadi* (natural divisions of time), *Vyadhyavastha* (stages of disease)
Anala (digestive capacity)	*Sama* (normal), *Tiksna* (acute), *Visama* (irregular), *Manda* (dull)
Prakrti (constitution)	*Vata*, *Pitta*, *Kapha*, *Vatapitta*,*Vatakapha*, *Pittakapha*, *Sama*
Vaya (age)	*Balya* (infancy), *Kaumara* (childhood), *Yauvana* (youth), *Vardhakya* (old age)
Sattva (mind)	*Sattvika* (calm), *Rajasika* (active), *Tamasika* (dull)
Satmya (habits)	*Okasatmya* (habituated by practice), *Desasatmya* (habituated by place), *Kulasatmya* (habituated by family)
Ahara (food)	*Dhanya* (grains), *Phala* (fruits), *Saka* (vegetables), *Harita* (spices and seasonings), *Mamsa* (meat), *Ksira* (dairy products), *Jala* (liquids), *Iksu* (sugarcane products)
Avastha (stages of disease)	*Sama-Nirama*, *Vega-Avega*, *Alpadosa-Bahudosa*, *Caladosa-Linadosa*

Thus the schemes for medical treatment are also holistic in their approach. The intention of treatment in all cases is to restore equilibrium. The purification of the body via the *pancakarma* is a distinctive feature, as are the promotive modes of treatment.

Table 2.4

Holistic Scheme for Treatment

Vyadhihara (curative)	*Langhana* (depletive)	*Sodhana* (purificatory)	*Vamana* (emesis), *Vireka* (purgation), *Vasti* (enemata) *Nasya* (errhines)[17], *Raktamoksa* (blood letting)
		Samana (restorative)	*Dipana* (activating digestive and metabolic process), *Pacana* (digestion and metabolism), *Ksut*, *Trt* (fasting), *Vyayama* (exercise), *Atapa* (exposure to sun), *Maruta* (exposure to wind)
	Brmhana (replenishing)	*Samana* (restorative)	*Snehana* (adding), *Stambhana* (saving)
Urjaskara (promotive)		*Rasayana* (restorative)	*Vatatapika* (casual)
			Kutipravesika (under controlled conditions)

Ayurveda only admits a drug into its materia medica when it has been rigorously appraised in terms of its biological properties and systemic action, classified into a therapeutic class, and fixed into a set of formulations and specifications provided for its processing and clinical application.

In this chapter we have tried to present the 'macrocosmic vision' of Ayurveda. Perhaps it is insufficient for making Ayurveda perfect or complete, although it has certainly contributed over the centuries to making Ayurveda a functional knowledge system. We hope that by reintroducing Ayurveda and showcasing its epistemology, we can inspire readers to truly open themselves to the implicit epistemologies that inform the several non-western knowledge system that exist today.

---

[17] Errhines: medication through nasal route in the form of drops, snuff, etc.

Bibliography

Dharampal (1971) *Indian Science and Technology in the Eighteenth Century*. Hyderabad: Academy of Gandhian Studies.

Needham, J. (1981) *Science in Traditional China — A Comparative Perspective.* Hong Kong: Chivere University.

Paradkar, B.H. (ed.) (1995) *Astanga Hrdayam.* Varanasi: Chaukhamba Prakashan.

Sharma, P.V. (1981) *Ayurveda History*. Varanasi: Chaukamba Prakashan. Second edition.

Sharma, P.V. (ed.) (1983) *Caraka Samhita,* Varanasi: Chaukhamba Prakashan.

Srinivas, M. D. (1986) An Indian Approach to Formal Logic and the Methodology of Theory Construction. *PPST Bulletin*, No.9, December.

Trikamji, Y. (ed.) (1992) *Susrutha Samhita.* Varanasi: Chaukhamba Prakashan. Fifth edition.

3

The Materia Medica of Ayurveda

P.M. Unnikrishnan

Traditional systems of medicine make use of a wide spectrum of natural resources as part of their pharmacopoeia. It is beyond the scope of this book to examine all the various systems and their use of these resources. But it is important to know how the resources are studied, the history of their use and the general principles by which they are incorporated into the respective pharmacopoeias. Significantly, the estimated 50,000 herbal formulations documented in Indian medical texts and used for a wide range of health conditions are about 10 times more than the 4,000-odd modern drugs that represent the sum total of the world's pharmacopoeia.

In this section, we focus on the importance given to medicinal plants and the concepts used to understand them as pharmaceutical material. Much of the information included here is drawn from Ayurveda and this will suffice to give an indication of how traditional systems work. However, in this context it is important to remember that each system is unique and based on differing principles. It is not always possible to apply generalisations drawn from Ayurvedic principles to all Indian traditional systems of medicine (local health tradition methodologies are quite distinct and will be examined in a subsequent chapter).

The use of plants for medicinal purposes has a very long and unbroken history in the Indian subcontinent. The *Ausadhi sukta* in the *Rig Veda*[18] is the oldest document available on medicinal plants in this region. It briefly describes the morphological character of medicinal plants, their habitat, their therapeutic classification and their uses in various ailments. Vedic hymns suggest that the use of plants for medication was initially based on observation of their effects on other species.

---

[18] *Rig Veda*, Section 10, Chapter 97, Verses 1-23.

Another important basis is sometimes referred to as the 'Doctrine of Signature'. Here, a part of the approach consisted of a comparison between plant parts and human body parts, such as hair, skin, blood and flesh. For example, there might be reference to the use of bark for skin conditions, *haridra* (turmeric) for jaundice, *laksa* and *manjista* (lac, *Rubia cordifolia* and other similar plants that were *red* in colour) for haemorrhage, etc.

There also appears to be a systematic documentation of the understanding of medicinal plants in the post-Vedic/Samhita[19] period, which came to be expressed in a body of knowledge called 'Ayurveda'. Ayurveda has a unique way of understanding plants — starting from the earliest Ayurvedic text available, the *Caraka Samhita* (1500 BC–400 AD), which provides an exhaustive description of around 600 plants and their medicinal uses. It contains much information related to nomenclature; descriptions for identification, biological properties and action; habitat; regional specifications of substitutes; and poisonous plants. The scripture also provides information on methods for collecting plants and of classifying, combining and processing their applications in specific stages and conditions, including incompatibility, contraindications, recipes and information regarding poisons. An important point that will become apparent as we proceed is that for Ayurveda, unlike Western science, classification and nomenclature serve different purposes.

There are a good number of classical Ayurvedic texts and manuscripts that deal with plants. These are largely *samhitas* (treatises), *samgrahas* (compendiums), *nighantus* (lexicons), *vyakhyas* (critical treatises) and texts on specific areas like pharmacy (*Bhaisajya kalpana*), paediatrics, etc. The major *samhitas* include *Caraka Samhita*, *Susruta Samhita*, *Astanga Samgraha* and *Astanga Hrdaya*, all of which were written before the seventh century. A few other treatises dating back to this period include the *Harita Samhita*, the *Bhela Samhita* and the *Kasyapa Samhita*, but these are not available in a complete form today.

---

[19] In historical descriptions the time frame has been roughly broken into four periods. We have adopted the same system here. The periods are the Vedic period (4000 BC - 1500 BC), the *Samhita* period (1500 BC – seventh century), the medieval period (eighth–fifteenth century) and the modern period (sixteenth century onwards). See *Ayurved Ka Vaijnanik Ithihas* by P.V. Sharma (1981). Varanasi: Chowkhambha Orientalia).

During the medieval period, or between the eighth and the fifteenth century, there have been many works written in the field of Ayurvedic pharmacology or *dravyaguna*, as it is called in Sanskrit. A good number of *nighantus* were coined during this period. These were appendices to the ancient *samhitas* and contain synonyms, qualities of drugs and the conditions in which they are to be used. (See Table 3.1 for the major *nighantus* and the period in which they are coined.)

Vyakhyas are critical commentaries on treatises and also carry elaborate references to plants. The important ones among them are *Ayurveda Dipika* by Cakrpanidatta for *Caraka Samhita* (11 AD), *Nyaya Candrika* by Gayadasa for *Susruta Samhita* (11 AD), *Nibandhasamgraha* by Dalhana for *Susruta Samhita* (12 AD), *Sarvanga Sundari* for *Astanga Hrdaya* by Arunadatta (13 AD), *Sasilekha* by Indu for *Astanga Samgraha* (13 AD), and *Tattvapradipika* by Sivadas Sen for *Caraka Samhita*.

The modern period saw works like *Bhavaprakasa Nighantu*, *Raja Nighantu*, *Saligrama Nighantu, Sivakosa, Vaidyavatamsam* and *Dravyagunasatakam* (seventeenth century.), *Rajavallabha nighantu* and *Nigahntu Ratnakaram* (eighteenth century) and the *Nighantu Samgraham* (nineteenth century).

Table 3.1 shows some of the important milestones in the history of Ayurvedic pharmacological literature and can be used as reference points for this chapter.

From this literature it is clear that the understanding of natural resources in the traditional pharmacopoeia had been quite dynamic. This knowledge was updated from time to time, for instance, with the study of new materials and the sharing of information between different cultures of medicine. Drugs whose identities have become obscure — such as *Asvavati*, *Somavati*, *Urjayanti*, *Udojas* — have been omitted. For instance, a group of plants called *Divyausadhi* that supposedly had powers similar to *soma*,[20] was included in the lists of the *samhita* period, but was later dropped by Vagbhata,

[20] *Divyausadhi* are celestial drugs mentioned in the *Susruta Samhita*. They have special therapeutic properties and fall into a group of rare drugs.

Table 3.1
Milestones in Ayurvedic Literature

Text name	Chronology	Author	Region of origin
Caraka Samhita	1500 BC – 400 AD	Agnivesa Caraka Drdhabla	Himalaya, Kashmir
Susruta Samhita	1500 BC – 500 AD	Susruta Nagarjuna	Kasi, Sindhudesa
Astanga Samgraha	500 AD	Vagbhata	Sindhudesa
Astanga Hrdayam	600 AD	Vagbhata	Sindhudesa
Astanga Nighantu	800 AD	Vagbhata	
Paryayaratnamala	900 AD	Madhava	Silahrada
Dhanvantari Nighantu	200 AD – 1000 AD	Unknown	Unknown
Cakradatta	1075 AD	Cakrpanidatta	Vangadesa
Dravyaguna samgraha	1075 AD	Cakrapanidatta	Vangadesa
Madhavadravyaguna	1250 AD	Madhava	Unknown
Sarngadhara Samhita	1300 AD	Sarngadhara	Devagiri
Nighantu Sesa	1200 AD	Hemacandra	Unknown
Siddhamantra	1210 AD –1247 AD	Kesava	Unknown
Hrdayadipaka Nighantu	1260 AD – 1271 AD	Bopadeva	Unknown
Madanapala Nighantu	1374 AD	Madanapala	Kasthanagara
Bhavaprakasa	1550 AD	Bhavamisra	Kasi, Kanyakubja
Bhavaprakasa Nighantu	1550 AD	Bhavamisra	Kasi, Kanyakubja
Raja Nighantu	1700 AD	Naraharipandita	Kasmira
Saligrama Nighantu	1896	Saligramvaisya	Muradabad
Siddhabhesajamanimala	1896	Krsnarama Bhatta	Jayapura

Source: Research Department, FRLHT.

the author of *Astanga Hrdaya* (600 AD), possibly because of the non-availability of the plants or due to difficulties in accessing them. Plants, the therapeutic properties of which were newly identified, were incorporated. There has been a gradual increase in the number of plants starting from the *Rig Veda* to the *Nighantus*; plants like *Sukanana*, *Parijata*, *Manaka*, *Mucukunda*, *Lataksturika*, *Virataru*, *Cakramarda*, *Mahanimba* and *Sakhota*, all of which were not found in *Caraka Samhita*, were later introduced by Susruta.

A number of drugs were introduced from other parts of the world through foreign contacts and trade and these have also been incorporated into the Ayurvedic therapeutic armoury. For instance, spices, aromatics and other drugs were exported while drugs like *hingu*, *kesara* and *madhuka* were imported. Exotic plants like brinjal, green chillies, potato, tapioca, tomato, pineapple, tea and coffee have been studied based on Ayurvedic parameters and incorporated into the literature only in the last few centuries.

In addition to Ayurvedic classifications, most of the books after Saligram Vaisya's *Saligramanighantu* (1896 AD) have tried to incorporate information from modern botany and pharmacognosy. Important works include the *Dravyaguna Samgraham* by Acharya Yadavjithrikamji, *Dravyagunavijnana* and *Priya Nighantu* by P.V. Sharma, and the *Nighantu Adarsa* by Bapalal Vaidya. These texts have also sought to incorporate drugs like *Gymnema sylvestre*, *Tylophora asthmatica*, *Peagnum harmal*, *Abroma angusta*, *Salacia oblonga*, and so on.

Professor P.V. Sharma description of the qualities of coffee (*Coffea arabica)*[21] is a good example of how a new plant is interpreted in terms of Ayurvedic concepts (see Table 3.2).

There are also a number of regional Ayurvedic works that explain the use of plants in different regions (ecosystems), which help us focus on past regional sensitivities. For example, a plant botanically known as *Salacia reticulata* is used for diabetic conditions in the Kerala tradition. This is documented in *Cikitsa Manjari*, which was probably written in the medieval

[21] *Dravyagunavijana* by P.V. Sharma (1981), Vol. 2. Varanasi: Choukhamba Bharati Academy.

Table 3.2

Qualities of *Coffea arabica* (Coffee)

Name	Coffee
Rasa	*Tikta*
Guna	*Laghu, ruksa*
Virya	*Usna*
Vipaka	*Katu*
Prabhava	*Hrdya*
Karma	*Jantughna, durgandhanasana, mutrala*
Dosakarma	*Kaphavata hara, pitta vardhaka*
Rogaghnata	*Jvara, svasa, kasa*

period, but no mention of this plant is found in mainstream texts. However, in more recent texts this plant has been incorporated under the name of *Saptacakra* (having seven whorls) and a group of synonyms like *Svarnamuli* (golden root), *Madhumehaghni* (anti-diabetic), etc., are now used to refer to it.

A large part of the information on plants is preserved through oral traditions or living *parampara*s (traditions) in various parts of the Indian subcontinent. There are also a number of manuscripts of which, unfortunately, many remain unpublished and un-researched even today. In his book, *Introduction to Dravyaguna*, Professor P. V. Sarma has listed nearly 230 manuscripts that focus exclusively on *Dravyaguna* and are preserved in various libraries the world over.[22]

It is interesting to note that the Ayurvedic system uses fewer drugs than the folk stream. This is probably due to the complexity of the studies needed to process and refine empirical experience and standardise it using Ayurvedic

[22] *Introduction to Dravyaguna* by P.V. Sharma (1976). Varanasi: Chaukhambha Orientalia.

parameters. Approximately 1,800 botanical species have been rigorously studied and incorporated in Ayurvedic literature, compared to around 8,000 species that are used in folk streams by various ethnic communities in different parts of the country.

How does Ayurveda actually build up its pharmacopoeia? An understanding of this will help us appreciate the rigorous criteria Ayurveda has developed for admitting a therapeutic substance into its materia medica.

Dravyagunavijnana is the special branch of Ayurveda that elaborates the qualities and biological actions pertaining to food and medicine. It covers the promotive, preventive and the curative applications of the plant drugs. Drugs are classified based on the source of origin as *audbhida* (plant), *jangama* (animal) and *parthiva* (mineral).

The word *osadhi* denotes herbaceous plants. The word *ausadha* in Sanskrit can be elaborated to mean '*oso daho dhiyate atraiti va*', i.e., a 'burning transformation resulting in a beneficial expression'. In other words, plants carry the creative energy that works on all life processes — especially all life transformations. *Osadhi* can be elaborated as '*osam rujam dhavati it*', i.e., 'one that removes pain'. Imbalances in the life process result in disease and any substance that regulates this process is called *ausadha*. Since plants constitute the major source of *ausadha*, the term '*ausadhi'* for them is appropriate.

Different parts and/or derivatives of a given plant source are used for particular conditions based on the understanding of their properties. After processing, these materials become *yoga* (combination). The word *ausadha* is used to denote the entity at all these three levels, i.e., the plant source, the plant part and the processed drug. The plant parts used by Ayurveda are root (*vilva)*, bark (*aragvadha*), heartwood (*khadira*), secretions (*fuggulu*), stalk (*palasa*), extracted juice (*vasa*), tender leaves *(amra*), alkali (*apamarga*), latex (*snuhi*), fruit *(amalaki*), flower (*japa*), ash (*narikela*), oil (*tila*), thorn (*salmali*), leaves (*karanja*), leaf buds (*nygrodha*), tubers (*surana*), sprouts (*mudga*), pedicle (*palasa*), petals (Lotus), stamen (*nagakesa*), seed (*vidanga*) and the whole plant (*durva*). The use of a few other parts like *limsaka* (internal skin), *paripotaka* (external skin) and *nirmoka* (scrapings) is less common.

Figure 3.1
Three-Tier Understanding of Ayurvedic Materia Medica

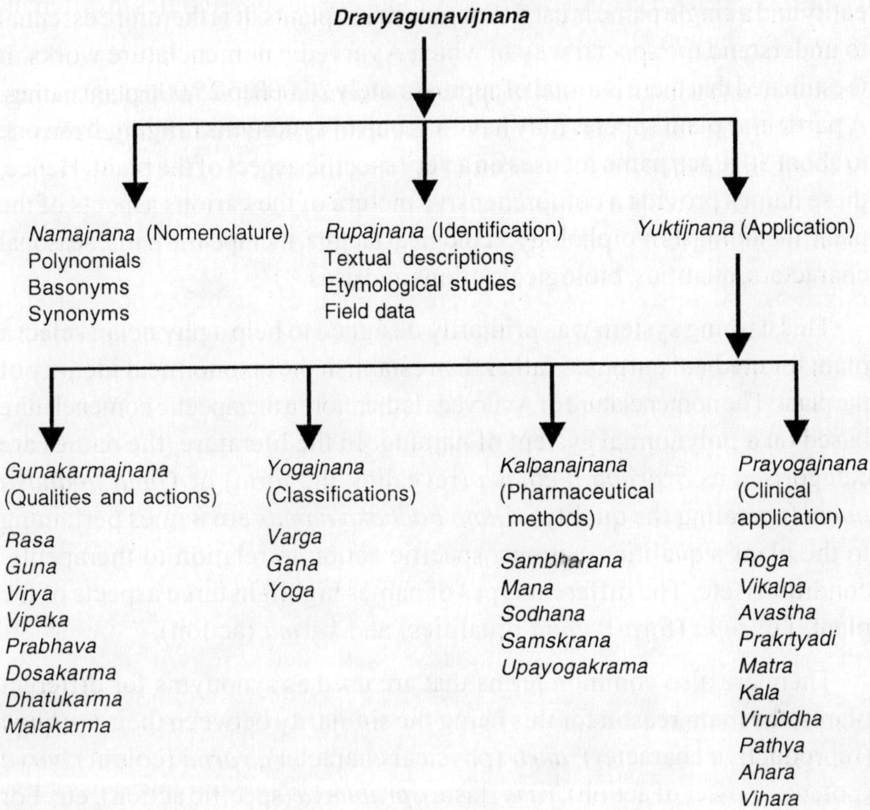

These materials are understood through a systematic, theoretical framework that is part of the *Dravyagunavijnana*. This is divided into the *Padarthavijnana* and the *Dravyavijnana*. *Padarthavijnana* is the science that deals with the study of the basic existential principles, i.e., *dravya* (substratum), *guna* (qualities), *karma* (actions), *samanya* (generic), *visesa* (specific) and *samavaya* (inherence). This knowledge provides an understanding of the dynamics of drug action. *Dravyavijnana* is the detailed pharmacology, which is divided into three subtopics, i.e., *nama* (nomenclature), *rupa* (identification) and *yuktijnana* (application). These constitute a three-tier understanding of *ausadha*.

The nomenclature of Ayurveda is not the binomial system that has been adopted by modern botany. In Ayurveda, there are many names for a single entity and a single name is used to denote many plants. It is therefore essential to understand the special way in which Ayurvedic nomenclature works. It is estimated that there is a total of approximately 20,000 to 25,000 plant names. A particular plant species may have a group of synonyms ranging from one to about 50. Each name focuses on a very specific aspect of the plant. Hence, these names provide a comprehensive picture of the various aspects of the plant, including its morphology, ecological factors, therapeutic parts, seasonal characters, qualities, biological actions and uses.

This naming system was primarily designed to help a physician select a plant for medical purposes rather than establish the taxonomical identity of the plant. The nomenclature of Ayurveda is therefore a therapeutic nomenclature based on a polynomial system of naming. In the literature, the names are categorised as *Svarupa bodhaka* (revealing the form) or *Guna bodhaka nama* (revealing the quality). *Guna bodhaka namas* are names pertaining to the plant's qualities, actions, specific action in relation to therapeutic conditions, etc. The different types of names highlight three aspects of the plant, i.e. *rupa* (form*), guna* (qualities) and *karma* (action).

There are also common terms that are used as synonyms for different plants, the main reason for this being the similarity between their *jatilinga* (reproductive character), *akrti* (physical character), *varna* (colour), *virya* (potency/power of action), *rasa* (taste), *prabhava* (specific action), etc. For example, the name *lata* is used as a synonym for *durva*, *manjista* and *priyangu* due to their common habitat. *Citra* is used for *urubuka, eranda* and *danti* due to their similarity in physical appearance; *sweta* for *surasa, katabhi, girikarnika and vaca* owing to their similarity in colour; *usana* for *marica* and *pippali* due to their similar potencies; *tikta* for *katurohini* and *kakatikta* because of their similar taste; and *amruta* for *guduci* and *haritaki* due to their similarity of biological action. From a string of such names (*nama mala*), a physician is easily able to position plants in the therapeutic context.

In order to gain a better understanding of the Ayurvedic nomenclature, let us consider the various meanings of the plant *Tinospora cordifolia*, which is known as *guduci* (one of several other synonyms) in Sanskrit. As we can see, its different synonyms provide us with comprehensive information about the plant. Based on its morphological characteristics, it is named *amrtavalli, amrtalata, somavalli, somalatika*, etc. The words *valli* and *lata* specify that it is a weak-stemmed plant. *Mandali, kundali nagakumari* and *tantrika* denote its circular form and its spread. *Cchadmika* indicates that it has thick foliage while *vatsadani* refers to the fact that its leaves are eaten by calves. Other synonyms that are in usage are *syama*, which means that its stem is of a smoky hue; *dhara*, which indicates that there are grooves on the stem; and *cakralaksana*, which refers to its wheel-like appearance when the stem is cut. *Cchinna, cchinnaruha, cchinnodbhava* and *cchinnangi* indicate the capacity of the cut stem to grow easily. All these synonyms fall under the category of *svarupa bodhaka nama*.

Among the synonyms that fall under the category *gunabodhaka nama*s of *guduci*, *amruta* indicates its nectar-like property. *Soma, rasayani, vayastha* and *jivanti* denote its action as an elixir and a strong rejuvenative. *Jvaranasini* and *jvarari* denote its anti-febrile activity.

This system of multiple names can be seen in local traditions as well. According to a Gujarati proverb '*Bar gauye boli badlaya*' (every 12 miles, the language or the dialect changes). According to *Dhanvanthari Nighantu*, a tenth century text, there are numerous regional names for plants and many of the classical names are coined from these. For example, grapes are called *dakh* in many north Indian languages and *draksa* in Sanskrit. *Gokharu* is called *goksura*, while *bhang* is *bhanga* in Sanskrit. *Muringa*, a South Indian name for drumstick, becomes *murungi* in Sanskrit. Further, the text claims that names are only meant for a practical purpose, i.e., for identification and usage.

Since a major portion of Ayurvedic literature is in Sanskrit, a comprehensive knowledge of the Sanskrit language is required for understanding the various aspects of Ayurvedic nomenclature. A single name can have different grammatical variants; for instance, the word *yasti* is used as *yastika*, *yastimadhu*, *yastimadhuka*, *yastyahva*, *yastyahvaya, yastyahvika, madhuyasti, madhuyastika*, etc. All these names pertain to the same entity and the root of the word does not change. In some cases, the gender of the words plays a very important role; for instance, the word *pippala* denotes *bodhivruksa* when used in the male gender, but in the female gender it denotes long pepper (*pippali*). Likewise, *mrnala* is lotus and *mrnali* is *lamajjaka* (touch-me-not). When the same word becomes *amrnala,* it denotes *usira*. All these aspects are described in detail in the Sanskrit lexicon, *Amarakosa*.

We can also gain a lot of insight into the medical aspects of plants if we analyse the terms etymologically. The same word may carry different shades of meanings (like the word *ausadha*). Additionally, there are many more grammatical issues that need thorough interdisciplinary research. According to a famous verse: '*Kanadam paniniyam ca sarva sastropakarakam*', meaning that the *sastras* expounded by Kanada and Panini, which include physics, metaphysics, epistemology, logic and the science of language, are the basis for all other *sastras* and are a prerequisite for an in-depth understanding of them.

Caraka Samhita says that the real expert on medicinal plants is one who, besides their nomenclature and identification, is also well versed in their applications, i.e., their qualities, actions and uses. It is mentioned that, properly used, even poison can become a good remedy; similarly, nectar can become poison if improperly used. The designing of an ideal drug (drug design needs a good understanding of a plant at four levels) involves several sophisticated factors. These are *gunakarma jnana* (knowledge of properties and actions), *yoga jnana* (knowledge of formulations), *kalpana jnana* (knowledge of preparations) and *prayoga jnana* (knowledge of applications). A deep understanding of incompatibilities is also necessary for the appropriate use (*samyak yoga*) of drugs. It is quite unfortunate that current practice seldom takes these factors into serious consideration. The design of most of the patented drugs available in the market today is very poor, as is the state of present-day Ayurvedic drug research.

The *guna karma* (qualities and actions) of a plant include *rasa* (taste), *guna* (qualities), *virya* (potency), *vipaka* (post-digestive effect), *prabhava* (specific effect), *karma* (action), *dosakarma* (action on dosa), action on *dhatu* (body tissues) and *mala* (waste products). To comprehend these, one has to know the *Panchmahabhuta* composition, i.e., the states of the five material principles of the plant.

Table 3.3

***Rasas* and their *Pancamahabhuta* Composition**

Madhura	*Amla*	*Lavana*	*Tikta*	*Katu*	*Kasaya*
Jala	*Agni*	*Prthvi*	*Vayu*	*Vayu*	*Vayu*
Prthvi	*Prthvi* (*Caraka*)	*Agni* (*Susruta*)	*Akasa*	*Agni*	*Prthvi*
	Agni	*Jala*			
	Jala (*Susruta*)	*Agni* (*Caraka*)			

Rasas (taste) are an important factor in evaluating the *bhoutika* (element) composition of a plant drug, which is determined by the effect of each *rasa* on the body. The *rasas* thus become the index of *bhoutika* composition and the drugs action on *tridosa*).

Digestion and metabolic processes play an important role in deciding the biological effect of a drug, because all drugs have to pass through the digestive cycle (*jathara*, *dhatu, bhutagni paka*). While the *bhoutika* composition of some drugs may continue unaltered even after digestion, in some cases it may be altered altogether in the course of its metabolism, and this change is reflected in *vipaka*. Thus, when there is more than one *rasa* in a particular *dravya*, the *vipaka* becomes a better index of its action.

Most of the drugs, e.g., *haritaki, amalaki, garlic, ginger, pippali* (Indian long pepper), have a broad spectrum of activity. The action of each substance is decided by its inherent potency. This is of two types: hot and cold. This potency can be modified by certain intrinsic factors that, after *rasa,* become a second index for the drug. These factors are called *gunas*. There are also 10 opposing qualities (*dvandva guna*), which are different from each other due to the relative preponderance of *mahabhutas*.

The biological activities of a plant that are not explained by these parameters (i.e., *rasa, guna, virya,* etc.) are attributed to a fourth, overriding parameter called *prabhava*. Even though it is mentioned that *prabhava* is *acintya* (that is, beyond inferential thought), scholars like Sharma have modified the term to *acintita* (unthought of).[23]

There are approximately 150 types of pharmacological actions (*karma*) listed in Ayurvedic literature. These are specific actions that the *dravya* exerts on the body through the different combinations of factors and can be classified into categories like *langhana* (depletion), *brmhana* (nourishing), *vamana* (emesis) and *virecana* (purgation).

The texts say that drug principles do not act solely because of the power of their qualities (*gunas*). The power of their physical nature (*Pancamahabhautic* composition) is equally important. But drugs act in a specific period of time after reaching a specific body substratum (*dhatu*), thus achieving a result that is very specific to each drug. What it achieves is called the drug action. The manner in which it acts depends on the *potency (virya)*. *Where* it acts is the 'target site', *when* it acts is the 'time of action', *how* it does is the *'stratagem'* and *what* it does is the 'final result' (*phalam*). The drugs thus act through the following factors: *dravya* (drug substance), *guna* (quality), *adhikarana* (substratum), *kala* (time), *yukti* (application), *artha* (means), *abhipreta* (intent), *karma* (action), *upaya* (stratagem) and, lastly, *phalam* (effect).

The second level of understanding is *yogajnana*, which includes grouping, classifying or formulating drugs. Classification or grouping of plants has a history dating back to the Vedic period. Elementary classifications group the plants into flowering and non-flowering, fruiting and non-fruiting, etc. This grouping is intended for therapeutic purposes as flowering or fruiting plants have definite therapeutic implications. Other classifications are based on *panca mahabhuta, tridosa, rasa, virya*, *karma*, etc. Based on these factors, drugs have been grouped into *varga* and *gana*. All *vargas* are primary, non-clinical, therapeutic classifications based on common morphological features, qualities and actions. This type of classification is mostly found in the

[23] *Introduction to Dravyaguna* by P.V. Sharma (1976). Varanasi: Chaukhambha Orientalia.

Table 3.4
***Guna* (Physical Properties)**

Guna	*Akasa*	*Vayu*	*Agni*	*Jala*	*Prthvi*
1 *Laghu* (light)	*	*	*		
2 *Guru* (heavy)					*
3 *Sita* (cold)				*	
4 *Usna* (hot)			*		
5 *Snigdha* (unctuous)				*	
6 *Ruksa* (dry)			*		*
7 *Manda* (slow)					*
8 *Tiksna* (sharp)			*		
9 *Sthira* (stable)					*
10 *Sara* (mobile)				*	
11 *Mrdu* (soft)	*			*	
12 *Kathina* (rough)					*
13 *Visada* (clear)	*	*	*		
14 *Picchila* (slimy)				*	
15 *Slaksna* (yielding)			*		
16 *Khara* (rough)		*			
17 *Suksma* (subtle)	*	*	*		

(contd.)

(Table 3.4 contd.)

Guna	*Akasa*	*Vayu*	*Agni*	*Jala*	*Prthvi*
18 *Sthula* (gross)					*
19 *Sandra* (dense)					*
20 *Drava* (fluid)				*	
Special *gunas*					
Suska (dry)		*	*		
Vyavayi (Visas)	*	*			

nighantus, even though *Brhatrayi*[24] also mention a few *vargas*. The *gana* is a more sophisticated, clinical, application-based classification given in the *samhitas*, which is used in the designing of drugs.

Plants are also organised into many drug formulations (around 50,000 in the classical texts) to suit specific diseases, disease types, stages and so on. These are specifically designed for easy, practical applications. According to the *Caraka Samhita*, many more such *yogas* can be designed by an in-depth application of the principles.

Siddhamantra, a text written 1210 AD, provides an elaborate classification based on *tridosa* and its various permutations. It includes nine *vargas* and 42 *upavargas* pertaining to approximately 650 drugs. The *Caraka Samhita* of 1500 BC explains the classification based on *rasas*: *madhura, amla, lavana, katu, tikta* and *kasaya skandhas*. In *Astanga Hrdaya*, this has been further elaborated into 64 groups, which are all permutations of these six *rasas*. *Abhidhanaratnamala* (*Sadrasa Nighantu,* probably written in the twelfth century) also classifies drugs based on taste. There are six

[24] *Brhatrayi* includes three major texts in Ayurveda — the *Caraka Samhita*, *Susruta Samhita* and *Astanga Hrdaya*.

chapters — *madhura* (102), *amla* (32), *lavana* (11), *tikta* (128), *Katu* (70) and *kasaya* (115) — which mention a total of 458 drugs.

Based on their clinical action, 50 *ganas* (basic formulations), such as *jivaniya*, *brmhaniya* and *bhedaniya*, have been mentioned in the *Caraka Samhita*. These are groups of 10 drugs each that have a specific function in common. Whereas in *Susruta Samhita* there are 37 groups, which only together act on a group of symptoms. These include *varunadi*, *aragvadhadi*, *eladi*, *vacadi*, *sarivadi* and so on. The peculiarity of this grouping is that each drug in a group has a specific role to play in a clinical application. It may serve as the main drug, an adjuvant or synergist, a corrective, a balancer or as a vehicle.

The other classifications include combinations like *Triphala* (three fruits), *Trikatu* (three spices), *Dasamula* (10 roots), *Pancakola*, *Caturjata*, *Pancatikta* (five bitters), *Panca pallava* (five tender leaves), *Astavarga* (a group of eight) and *Trimada* (three intoxicants). These are well-designed combinations that have wide-ranging therapeutic applications. For instance, in the group called *Triphala* (three fruits), *Haritaki* has a very efficient action on the *srotas* (body channels), *amalaki* on *agni* (the transformative principle) and *vibhitaki* on *dhatu* (body tissues). This combination is thus used in a variety of clinical conditions.

Food substances have been grouped in the literature into different *vargas* like *dhanya* or grains (*suka dhanya*, *sami dhanya*, *ksudradhanya), saka varga* or vegetables (*puspa*, *patra*, *phala*, *nala*, *kanda*), *phala varga* (fruits) and *taila varga* (oils).

The knowledge of combining individual drugs to make a formulation is called *yogajnana*. Different factors, such as drug incompatibility, drug interaction and potency, are taken into consideration here. The drugs are also combined to facilitate a synergistic action. A compound formulation usually has the following components — a main drug, adjuvants, balancing drugs and a vehicle.

There are mainly three types of incompatibilities — of proportion (*mana*), of quality (*guna*) and of action (*karma*). Honey and ghee in equal proportions should not be mixed and taken internally. This is an example of the first kind of incompatibility. Drugs with different *rasas,* for example *virya* and *vipaka*, are incompatible qualitatively. Similarly, materials like radish should not be combined with a drug with an opposite action, such as that of *dhataki,* which is '*karma virodha*'. The incompatible food or drug may cause serious skin diseases, fistula, anaemia, haemorrhagic disorders, oedema, etc.

Ayurveda also mentions that, in principle, there is nothing in the universe that is non-medicinal. There is a famous story that illustrates how open-ended it is. Jivaka, a renowned physician during the period of the Buddha, was asked by his guru to fetch some herb that was non-medicinal. He travelled the entire length and breadth of the country but could not find anything that was not medicinal: every plant he saw had some medicinal use and so he returned empty-handed. Thus Jivaka was recognised as a great physician. This gives a good picture of the richness of the medicinal flora and an understanding of their use during that period.

Classification of habitat (*desa vikalpa*), instructions for collection (*samgrahana viddhi*), storage, measurements (*mana*), purification of materials, details of food substances and poisons are a few other topics that are covered in the available literature.

According to Caraka, a classification system is required to understand the ideal habitat (*desa*) for collection of a drug as well as its ecological variations. Habitats are thus divided into *jangala* (dry land), *anupa* (wetland) and *sadharana* (moderate land). A separate classification based on *pancamahabhuta* has also been provided. The types of vegetation to be found in each *desa* have been grouped and the peculiarities of each in relation with the body physiology elaborated. *Jangala desa* is dry land and contains plants like *kadara, khadira, asana, asvakarna, sala, sami, somavalka, kakaubha,* and *simsapa*. *Anupa desa* is wet or marshland and contains *hintala*, *narikela*, *Kadali*, *Tamala*. The *sadharana desa* has a mixture of species belonging to both the *jangala* and *anupa* classifications.

The instructions for collection include information on the parts that should be collected, the astrological specifications, the best locations, the accompanying rituals and chanting and the seasonal specifications. For instance, it is advised that the raw drugs should not be collected from graveyards, from the vicinity of slaughterhouses, from gardens, anthills, main roads, religious places, markets

Table 3.5

Seasons and the Collection of Drugs

Parts to be collected	Season
Leaves, branches	Spring, monsoon
Root	Summer or late winter
Stem bark, tuber, latex	Autumn
Heartwood	Early winter
Fruit, flower	According to availability

Source: *Caraka Samhita.*

and garbage pits. The reasons for this may be many, such as hygiene, conservation, potency or efficacy.

There is also an important relationship between the collecting of drug substances and the seasons (see Table 3.5).

Each part of a plant has a particular *pancamahabhuta* composition and is administered during a specific season, condition or stage of the disease. For instance, in *netra chikitsa prakarana* (treatment of eye diseases), many of the single-drug recipes contain flowers, tender leaves and fruits. The eye is an organ which is equally susceptible to both *kapha* and *pitta dosa*. These plant parts are *laghu* (light) and *snigdha* (unctuous), and are primarily composed of *tejomahabhuta*, which can alleviate some these conditions.

Plants or their parts are collected during seasons that they grow to maturity (become *paka).* Since seasonal manifestations are not the same in every region, there are differences of opinion among authors regarding the seasons for collection. Instructions for collection are also found for plants with specific *virya* or *karma*, as, for example, 'for the purposes of emesis and purgation the drug should be collected in late winter'. Drugs that need to be collected in their fresh state (e.g., *guduci, vasa, satavari,* etc.) and those whose power is enhanced after being stored for more than one year (e.g., *vidanga, krsna* — black pepper and *dhanya* — coriander) come with separate instructions.

Other interesting information includes substitutes (*Pratinidhi dravya*) and the quantities in which they can be used when the suggested drug is not available, viz., *satavari* for *meda* and *mahameda*, *vidari* for *jivaka,* and *rsabhaka* and *musta* for *ativisa*.

Pharmaceutical preparation (*kalpanajnana*) is another area that is extensively elaborated in Ayurvedic literature. During the pre-Vedic period, pharmaceutical preparations were limited to fresh juices, pastes, etc. More elaborate documents regarding pharmacy and appliances are available from the *Rig Vedic* period. A very systematic presentation of pharmacy is available in the *Samhitas*. Some treatises have separate sections called *kalpasthanas* that are devoted solely to pharmaceutical preparations. Having multiple *kalpana* (forms of medicine) is one of the qualities of an ideal drug. Ayurveda contains approximately 70 to 80 varieties of preparations of drugs and food supplements.

According to the *Caraka Samhita*, there are five primary pharmaceutical preparations — *svarasa* (juice), *kalka* (paste), *srta* (decoction), *sita* (cold infusion) and *phanta* (hot infusion) — with their potency decreasing in successive order. From these five derive a variety of *kalpanas*, numbering more than 70. *Ghrta* (medicated ghee), *taila* (medicated oil), *gutika* (tablet), *curna* (powder), *leha* (linctus), *arista* and *asava* (fermented preparation) and *panaka* (syrup) are a few of them. The food preparations include different varieties of *peya* (gruel), *supa* (soups), *apupa*, *pupalika* (cakes), as well as fermented drinks like *varuni, prasanna, jagala* and *kadambari.*

The drug is processed for refinement and potentiation, as well as for compatibility with the bio-assimilation mechanism and receptivity of the host. It is also meant to extract and retain the active fraction to make it maximally effective. There are multiple processes involved in the preparation, such as *aditaya paka* (cooking in sun light), *apakarsana* (elimination), *jarjarikarana* (disintegration) *tapana* (heating), *dahana* (burning), *dhupana* (fumigation) and *bhavana* (impregnation). A detailed description of the process, technology and instruments required is also available. The methodology for purifying drugs is also explained.

As clinical application is the most important purpose (*prayojana*) of Ayurveda, it has been explained in great detail. *Prayogajnana* is thus concerned with dosage, adjuvants, dietary restrictions and the time of consumption. Information on how to select drugs on the basis of the individual's constitution, disease type and stage of disease is provided, along with precise dosages for every drug. Also included are details about contraindications for several drugs. For instance, it is advised that drugs like ginger should not be taken in the case of bleeding disorders, skin disorders, anaemia and during summer and autumn. Similarly, those who are tired, weak, lean or exhausted due to fasting should avoid *haritaki*, as should individuals with a *pitta* constitution, pregnant women and persons with bleeding disorders. When one uses plants like *tuvaraka* or *aruskara*, hot water should not be taken along with them. Eight types of incompatibilities have been mentioned in the context of contraindications (*viruddha*).

Another important aspect of the traditional medical pharmacopoeia is its spiritual dimension. The spiritual dimension of medicinal plants is implicit in their existence. Ayurveda has evolved from a profound cultural and philosophical perspective that is also shared by other Indian *sastras*. According to the *Samkhya* school there are two aspects of creation — the manifest (*prakrti*), which is expressed as a combination of matter and form, and the unmanifest (*purusa*), which is formless. In this conception, the unmanifest and the manifest are two sides of the same coin and therefore represent a continuum on which consciousness (*cetana*) and matter exist in the same way as energy exists on a continuum with matter.

So far, we have focused on plants by way of showing how the materia medica of Ayurveda works, but it must be remembered that other materials are also used in the Ayurvedic pharmacopoeia. While plant resources do form the major portion of the pharmacopoeias, metals, minerals and animal products are also used.

In Ayurveda, 15 to 20 per cent of the materia medica comprises of animal, animal products and processed substances. *Caraka Samhita* mentions 230

Figure 3.2
Plant, Animal, Metal and Mineral Usage in Ayurveda in the Medieval Period

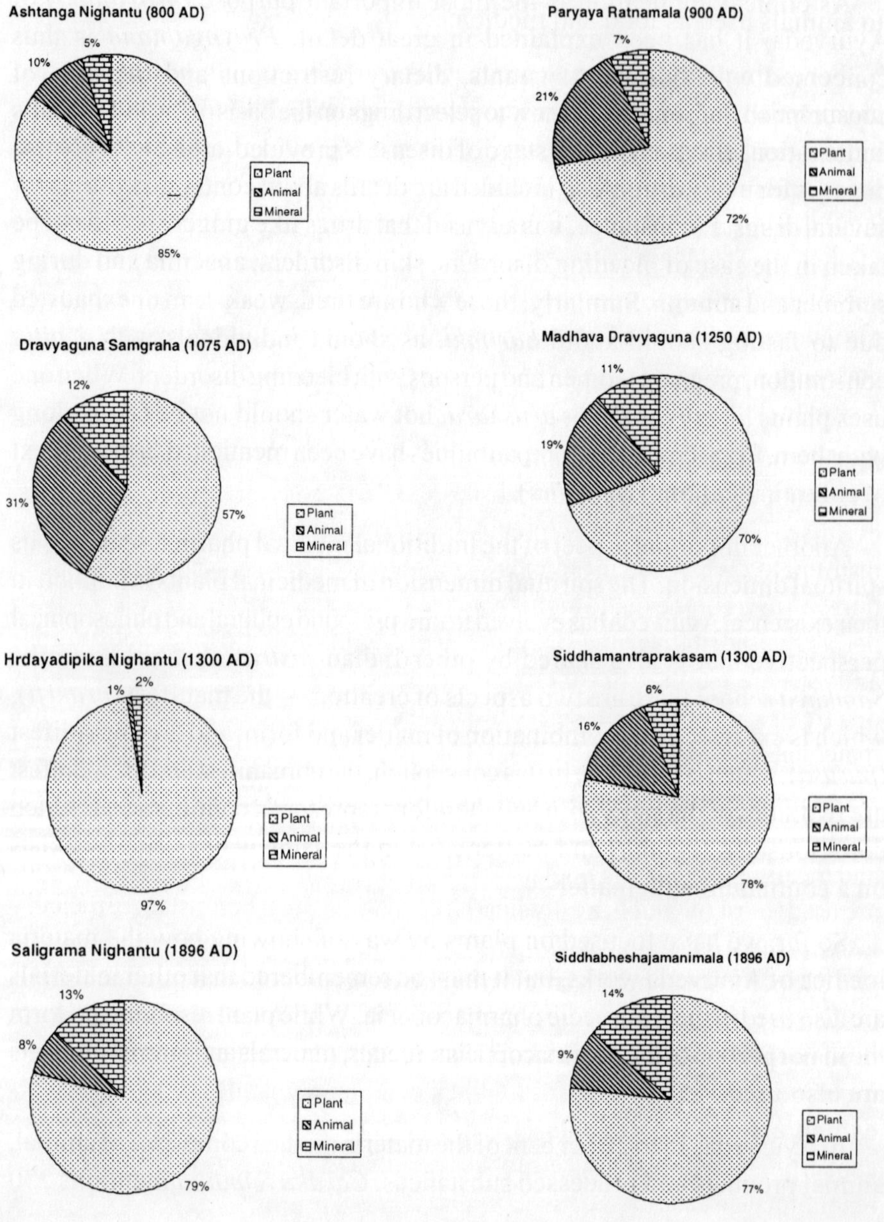

types of animals and 380 types of animal substances while the *Susruta Samhita* contains information regarding 225 types of animals. *Kasyapa Samhita* has 400 references to 256 types of animal substances, the majority of which pertain to animals used as food and medicine.

For example, milk and milk products like curd, buttermilk, butter, ghee and cream are all found in the Ayurvedic pharmacopoeia. Milk, whether of the cow, buffalo, goat, sheep, elephant, camel, donkey or the human being, has medicinal uses. Buttermilk is commonly used in haemorrhoids, urinary disorders, diabetic conditions, irritable bowels, spleen disorders, vomiting and obesity. Honey is also widely used in Ayurveda, especially as a carrier for several drugs. By itself, honey is used to treat obesity, diabetic conditions, hiccoughs, respiratory afflictions, diarrhoea, thirst as a pathological condition, worm infestation and poisoning.

Animals are also used in the extraction process. Leeches (*jaluka*) are used for the extraction of impure blood from the body as well as for abdominal swellings, piles, inflammatory abscess, skin diseases, rheumatoid arthritis, eye diseases and poisonous bites. Certain animal parts are used for making instruments, which aid in diagnosis and surgery. The instruments are divided into *yantras* (blunt instruments) and *sastras* (sharp instruments). *Yantras* derive their form from the shape of the mouth of different birds and animals and thus are named after them. Horns of different animals, such as of the ox, are used for bloodletting. Animal tendons and hair are used as suturing materials.

Ayurveda includes *Rasasastra* — the science of metal and mineral medicine. The *Rig Veda* and the *Atharva Veda* have mentioned minerals and metals that have potential use as medicine. About 60 minerals and metals are used, most of which are obtained from natural ores. For instance, mercury is extracted from cinnabar (*hingula*), while iron is extracted from iron pyrite and copper from copper pyrite. Alkaline earth metals, such as conch shells (*shankha*) and cowries (*kapardika*), which are obtained from the sea, are used in their entirety. Heavy metals like mercury and lead are used in the metalo-organic complex. Most of the metals and minerals used in Ayurveda exhibit anti-ageing actions, as well as help to increase virility and brain capacity. They are also used to treat leucoderma, typhoid, epilepsy, and respiratory diseases.

While we have dealt only with Ayruveda in this chapter, it is important to remember that there are other traditional medical systems like *Siddha* and *Unani*, which also have a rich repository of knowledge and classificatory systems. Though a detailed examination of these codified systems is beyond the scope of this book, we will look at the folk traditions in later chapters.

Bibliography

Ramanathan, A.A (1983) *Amara kosa*. Madras: Adayar Library. Vol 1-3.

Publication Department, (1985) *Dravyagunavijnanam*. Vol. 2. Thiruvananthpuram: Ayurveda College.

Krishnamurthy, K. H. (1991) *A Sourcebook on Indian Medicine*. New Delhi: D.K. Publishers.

Rammanohar, P. (1994) *Nomenclature Taxonomy of Vrksayurveda*. Coimbatore: Lok Svasthya Parampara Samvardhan Samithi.

Sharma, P. V. (ed.) (1992) *History of Indian Medicine*. Delhi: Indian National Science Academy.

Sharma, P. V. (1981) *Dravyagunavijana*. Varanasi: Choukhamba Bharati Academy.

4

Building a Bridge Between Local Health Cultures and Codified Traditions

A.V. Balasubramaniam

As has been mentioned earlier, a major objective of this book is to introduce the reader to a wide spectrum of health practices prevalent in India. We have looked at Ayurveda as one form of the codified tradition. We have also had a brief look at the folk tradition. What we need to look at now is the symbiotic relationship between the two. The chapter attempts to not merely describe local traditions but, with a few examples, to also understand and explain them in the light of the theory and principles of the codified Indian systems of medicine (ISM).

Rationale Underlying Some Common Local Practices

Disease/condition: Diarrhoea

Treatment (a): Greens should be avoided and buttermilk and rice should be taken (reported from localities in Tamil Nadu in the 'Mother and Child Health Survey').[25]

Rationale: In diarrhoea, the *jatharagni*, i.e., digestive power, is not normal and its action is diminished. Greens are not advised as they are *guru*, i.e., difficult to digest. Buttermilk (*takram*) and rice, on the other hand, have the qualities of *dipana* (appetiser or that which increases the digestive fire) and *kasaya rasa* (astringent taste). It is said in *Astanga Hrdaya* (*Sutra sthana*, Chapter 5) that *takram* is light (to digest), has a *kasaya* (astringent) and *amla* (sour) taste, and because of this it improves appetite and controls *kapha* and *vata*.

---

[25] Survey on Traditional Practices of Mother and Child Health in the Districts of Chengalpet and Villupuram conducted by Patriotic and People Oriented Science and Technology Foundation (PPST), Madras, in 1998.

Disease/condition: Scorpion bite

Treatment: If bitten by a scorpion, leaves of *ber* (*Zizyphus jujuba*) and *haridra* (*Cucurma longa*) should be put in a pot over a fire and the smoke inhaled by the person bitten reported in rural areas around Varanasi.[26]

Rationale: The symptoms of poisoning by a scorpion's bite are inflammation of the tongue, fever, loss of power of the sense organs, perspiration, fainting and dryness of the mouth. The smoke, when inhaled, acts as a stimulant. *Ber* possesses the qualities of *pittasamaka* and *trsnanivarana* (controller of *pitta* and reliever of thirst). As the *Bhavaprakasa Nigantu* (*Haritakyadi varga, sloka* 77) says: "*Bhedhyagni krt sarvam laghu, trsna klamasrajit,*" i.e., *ber* improves *agni*, the quality of *rasa* and *rakta* and also cures *rakta vikaras* and fatigue.

Disease/condition: Eye ailment(s)

Treatment: For conjunctivitis, make a solution with dried *dhanyakam* (*Coriandrum sativum*) and cold water and put a drop in each eye before retiring at night (reported by *dais* [midwives][27] in the villages of Haryana).

Rationale: *Dhanyakam* is described in the *Bhavaprakasa Nigantu* (*Haritakyadi varga, sloka* 87-88) as *madhura rasa* (sweet) and *grahi* (astringent). It controls *daha* (burning sensation) and *krmi* (infection) and is said to be helpful in cases of *Netrabhisyanda* (conjunctivitis) and *Netra vrana* (ulcers in the eye/corneal ulcers).

Madras: Local beliefs

A survey of food habits in Madras in the 1960s[28] revealed several traditional beliefs relating to food. Some of these are:

- Milk, egg, chicken soup, goat's leg soup, fish and oily foods are to be taken for asthma.

[26] *Traditional Healers in Community Health* by K. P. Shukla (1981). Varanasi: Gomathi Krishna Publications.

[27] *Dais – the Traditional Birth Attendants in Village India* by D.N. Kakar (1980). New Delhi: New Asian Publishers.

[28] A Survey of Nutrition Habits of Elderly Persons in Madras State (1965–67) conducted by the Dr A. Lakshmipathi Research Unit, Nagarjun (1969) Vol. XII, No. 8, pp. 35-52.

- Fish, milk, fruits, flesh, garlic, onion, liver soup, crab, fenugreek, *krsna jiraka* (*Nigella sativa*), *vidari* (*Ipomoea digitata*), etc., are prescribed to increase the secretion of milk.

Classical description

1 All food items prescribed for asthma have the qualities of *brmhana* (bulk promoting, nutritional, increasing *rasadidhatus*) and *vatahara.* Asthma (*Tamaka svasam*) is an emaciating disease caused by vitiated *vata* — thus the *gunas* of milk, egg, etc., act against the causative factors by controlling *vata.*

2 All the items mentioned in this list are *Brmhana* (bulk promoting), *Vrsya* (aphrodisiac) and *Sapta dhatu vardhaka* (assisting the formation of the seven body tissues). The last one — *vidari* — is a very good emenogogue. It is said in the *Bhavaprakasa Nigantu* (*Guducyadi varga, slokas* 191, 192): *"Vidari madhura snigdha brmhani stanya sukrada sita svarya mutrala ca jivani balavarnada guruh pittasra pavana dahan hanti rasayani"*, i.e., *vidari* is sweet, unctuous and bulk promoting, and improves breast milk and semen. It cools the body, improves the voice, assists in the formation of urine, and is life promoting. It also improves one's strength and complexion; lastly, it is heavy to digest, controls *pitta, rakta, vata* and burning sensation.

An essential aspect of disease prevention is the knowledge of *Rtucarya*. There are a number of practices that involve the adoption of certain food habits, etc., based on particular seasons or change of seasons. Some of these are in the nature of cultural practices. For example, it can be observed in many parts of India that the types of food eaten in winter generally tend to be heavier and more difficult to digest (in Ayurvedic terms *guru*) than foods eaten in summer, which tend to be lighter and easier to digest (in Ayurvedic terms *laghu*). This is in keeping with the Ayurvedic understanding that *agni*, which is responsible for our digestion, is more powerful during the cold winter months than during the hot summer months, when it is much weaker.

Other aspects include guarding against certain types of diseases that may be more prevalent in a given season. For example, it is customary in many parts of Andhra Pradesh to partake of preparations containing *neem* leaves and flowers (*nimba kusuma bhaksanam*) at the onset of *Vasanta rutu* (spring) and to continue taking it for the entire season. The theory behind this quite logical: the *kapha dosa* gets vitiated in *Vasanta rutu* and neem leaves serve as a corrective measure.

While local health practices in different parts of India are believed to have an independent 'genesis' from that of the codified knowledge systems like Ayurveda, Siddha, *gso-rig-pa* (Tibetan) and Unani, over time they have interacted with codified knowledge and have both influenced it as well as been influenced by it. The references given below from *Caraka Samhita* and *Susruta Samhita* testify to their relationship.

Local health practices are also extremely diverse. They have been invented or discovered by different local cultures in the course of their interaction with their immediate natural environment and in response to local needs. They therefore use plant, animal and mineral resources that are ecosystem specific and their health practices are usually community specific. The degree of their theoretical sophistication depends on the nature of the local culture; generally, however, local practices seek to solve local problems without trying to provide general or universal solutions. For instance, the local health practices of Thakur tribals of the Western Ghats are different from those of the tribals of the northeast, and those of the shepherd communities (*Dhangars*), who dwell in the plains of Maharashtra, are different from those of shepherd communities in Rajasthan. Again, the local health practices of the rural *Brahmins* of Tanjore are different from those of the *Chettiars* who live in the same region, because both these communities have very different lifestyles.

Historical Backdrop

It is interesting to note from historical sources that certain areas boasted a very rich heritage of local health practices. A nineteenth-century survey gives us some idea about the number of local health practitioners, the largest categories among them being *dais* and snake doctors. This is in reference to parts of Bengal.[29]

---

[29] *Indian Science and Technology in the Eighteenth Century* by Dharampal (2000), Mapusa, Goa: Other India Press.

The survey speaks of two categories of physicians, of whom some were educated in Sanskrit, while others relied on Bengali translations. It says:

> The only difference that one has been able to discover between the educated and uneducated class of native practitioners is that the former prescribe with greater confidence and precision from the original authorities (medical texts), and latter with greater doubt and uncertainty from loose and imperfect translations.

It may come as a surprise to us that the practitioners surveyed included "31 smallpox inoculators"!

One practice about which very little is known even today is the traditional Indian method of inoculation against smallpox.[30] This fact might well pose a challenge to the recent claim that it is Western biomedicine that has eradicated smallpox from India. Inoculation against smallpox seems to have been widespread in large parts of northern and southern India before the eighteenth century. While one can find various references to this practice in the available literature, the description provided by J. Holwell, FRS, is perhaps one of the most detailed. He described the practice as he observed it in Bengal in 1767.[31]

Traditional Smallpox Inoculation in Bengal

Inoculation is performed by a particular tribe of *Brahmins* who are dedicated annually for this service from the different colleges over various provinces. They travel in small groups (of 3 or 4) from place to place so, as to reach various places some weeks before the usual onset of the disease. In Bengal, the inoculators normally arrive in February (or some times as late as March), before the onset of summer. The residents of each locality know the usual time when they arrive and observe a strict regimen for a month in advance. This consists of abstaining for a month from fish, milk and ghee.

---

[30] *Indian Science and Technology in the Eighteenth Century: Some Contemporary European Accounts* by Dharampal, (1983), Hyderabad: Academy of Gandhian Studies. Reprint.

[31] *An Account of the Manner of Inoculating for the Smallpox in the East Indies* by J. Z. Holwell (1767). London: Becket and de Hondt.

When they begin to inoculate, they pass from house to house and inoculate only those who have observed the regimen. Usually they inoculate outside of the arm midway between the wrist and elbow for the males and between the elbow and the shoulder for the females. Before the inoculation, the inoculator takes a piece of cloth in his hand and rubs the part to be inoculated for eight to ten minutes. He then makes a small prick with a small instrument till a drop of blood appears. After that he opens a linen double cloth and takes from there a small piece of cotton charged with various matter which he moistens with a few drops of Ganges water and applies it to the wound with a bandage. This remains in place for about six hours. The prohibition of fish, milk and ghee extends for one month from the day of inoculation.

Dr Holwell goes on to say: "When the before recited treatment is strictly followed, it comes as a miracle to hear that one in million fails of receiving the infection or of one that miscarries under it."

Some time around then, Dr E. Jenner had produced from the cow a vaccine for inoculation against smallpox. In 1804, the Superintendent General of Vaccine Inoculation banned the practice of traditional inoculation.[32] After the imposition of British rule in India, the fiscal system began to collapse. Various categories of specialists and functionaries who were maintained by the public system were thrown out and left to fend for themselves. The frequent smallpox epidemics, which were rampant in India during the nineteenth and early twentieth century, may be largely traced to the indifference of the state in making the required arrangements for universal vaccination on the one hand, and banning the traditional practice on the other.

Local Health Traditions of Surgery

Many of us are used to thinking of surgery as a highly sophisticated procedure that was made possible only in recent times by the advent of modern methods. It may therefore come as a surprise to know that there have been various local traditions of surgery and surgical techniques. Some of the areas in which these techniques are known to have existed are obstetrics, ophthalmology and even plastic surgery.

[32] *Report on the Progress of Vaccine Inoculation in Bengal 1802-3* by John Shoolbred (1804). Calcutta: East India Company Press.

There is considerable evidence in the medical as well as the *Dharmasastra* texts to indicate that Caesarean section — that is, the incision of the abdominal wall and uterus to deliver a child at the natural time of birth (or near the natural time of birth) — has been practised in India from very ancient times. The practice has been described in certain *Dharmasastra* texts (such as the *Baudhayana Pitrmedhasutra* and the *Vaikhanasa Grhyasutra*) as well as in the *Susruta*. Some observers, both in the nineteenth and twentieth centuries, have reported live children born by the performance of Caesarean section.

It is now also known that there used to be local traditions of surgical treatment of cataract. Dr Helenus Scott, who reported to the Royal Society of England on a variety of scientific practices, which he observed in India, wrote in 1792 to the President of the Royal Society:

> They practise with great success the operation of depressing the crystalline lens when it became opaque and from time immemorial they have cut for the stone at the same place which they now do in Europe.[33]

But it is perhaps in the area of plastic surgery that Indian traditions were the most advanced from the earliest times and had a profound influence on the practice of the art in various parts of the world.[34] The first detailed description of surgical replacement of the nose is found in *Susruta Samhita*. The two early methods practised in India — namely, the cheek flap method and the median forehead flap method — are still used by modern surgeons. The method of total nasal reconstruction was practised by the caste of brick makers and potters. The use of the forehead flap method has been in vogue in Maharashtra at least since the fifteenth century. There are also families of *Kangra* who are skilled in this art and the last surviving member of these families (Hakim Dinanath, who belongs to the potter caste) performed this

[33] *Aspects of Technology in Western India* consists of extracts from letters addressed from Bombay by Dr H. Scott to Sir Joseph Banks, President of Royal Society, London, between 1790 and 1801. See also *Indian Science and Technology in the Eighteenth Century* by Dharampal (2000). Goa: The Other India Press.

[34] 'The Impact of Indian Methods of Total Nasal Reconstruction' by C.S. Nichter, R.F. Margan and M.A. Nichter (1983). *Clinics in Plastic Surgery,* Vol.10, No.4 (October), pp. 635-47.

operation during the twentieth century. The publication of a report on the Indian method (of total nasal reconstruction) by British observers in 1794 aroused much interest in the West.

In contemporary times there is no detailed information regarding the prevalence of any traditional practices in surgery, though in some areas, such as in dentistry and ophthalmology, some traditions still survive.

Folk Knowledge and Classical Textual Knowledge

The prevalence of a large number of proverbs in local cultures in such diverse areas as agriculture and medicine is very important since they symbolise the nature of local knowledge. They contain the wisdom of thousands of years of experience. It is interesting to know the relative importance or status assigned to such 'folklore' in our tradition. While in any given area (such as medicine) there may exist a body of experts or learned professionals who have specialist knowledge, there are also other forms of local knowledge that are more diffuse or scattered amongst people who have their own remarkable systems of 'oral' transmission.

It is widely believed in the Indian tradition that, whatever the discipline, knowledge can and does prevail in various forms and also gets communicated in many ways, with each form serving its own purpose. For example, songs and literary works are classified in five groups based on how they are formulated and how comprehensible they are. These are *Narikelapakam, Iksupakam, Kadalipakam, Draksapakam* and *Ksirapakam*. The form most difficult to comprehend is the *Narikelapakam*, which has been likened to a coconut; to be eaten, the shell must be broken, the fruit grated and then mixed with food. *Iksupakam* has been compared to the sugarcane, which has to be crushed to extract juice. *Kadalipakam* is like the banana, which just has to be peeled before it is eaten. Even easier to comprehend is the *Draksapakam,* which is like the grape that can be eaten without any processing. However, the easiest form of all is the *Ksirapakam*, which is like milk that can be easily consumed and is a wholesome food for people in all age groups and in all conditions.

Similarly, literary compositions in Sanskrit are classified into three groups: *Prabhu Samhita, Suhrt Samhita* and *the Kantha Samhitha*. *Prabhu Samhita* instructs like a *prabhu* or master who punishes when rules are transgressed (e.g., instructions such as in the Vedas); *Suhrt Samhita*, which instructs like a friend who advises on what to do and what not to do (e.g., the *Puranas*); and the *Kantha Samhitha*, which instructs like a *kantha* or one's beloved, who cites examples, coaxes, pleads or persuades (as the situation may warrant) to achieve the same end, namely, '*Upadesa*' (as in *Kavyam*).

It is noteworthy that these different formulations or forms of communication are not understood as being part of a hierarchical system where one can replace or supersede another. Nor is any one of them considered the generally superior form. Each serves a specific need and may be the most appropriate for a particular context or a given purpose.

The general picture that emerges seems to be that the 'classical texts' in any area of learning may set out broad, general principles as well as illustrate their applications in different contexts. But in various regions local prescriptions are also available. These are based on the given situation and do not attempt to provide any generalities.

Relationship Between ISM and Local Traditions

The *Caraka Samhita* states (*Sutra sthana*, Chapter I, *sloka* 120–21) that: "*Ausadhir nama rupabhayam, janantehyajapavane, avipascaiva gopasca ye ca anye vanavasinah*" (the goatherds, shepherds, cowherds and other forest dwellers know the drugs by name and form). Similarly, *Susruta* states (*Sutra sthana*, Chapter 36, *sloka* 10) that – "*Gopalastapasa vyadha ye canye vana carinaha, mulaharasca ye tebhyo bheshaja vyaktirisyate*" (one can know about the drugs from the cowherds, *tapasvis*, hunters, those who live in the forest and those who live by eating roots and tubers).

A classical text such as the *Caraka Samhita* expounds general principles of drug action based on the six factors of *dravya, guna, rasa, virya, vipaka* and *prabhava*. It also discusses remedies for several diseases and lists specific drugs. These may get modified to suit local conditions. In any recipe for a drug, one can substitute a non-principal component (*apradhana dravya*) with an equivalent. This equivalent may be listed in the *sastras* or selected on the basis of the principle of *rasa, virya*, etc. From time to time, in tune with such an understanding, *vaidyas* produce regional texts and manuals that set out prescriptions for drugs in any given area based on what is available and suitable to the requirements of that area. For example, the text *Rajamrganka* lists 129 recipes and in his foreword, the editor — *Ayurvedacarya* (belonging to Tamil Nadu) — says that since the raw material is readily available, these recipes are not only easy to formulate but are also most suited to the area. This is in accordance with *Caraka*'s dictum that: "For a person who belongs to a particular country or a region, *ausadhis* from the same region are most wholesome."

The fact that it is the particularity of the context that is the overriding consideration and that the *sastric* principles are to be considered as precepts and guidelines and not applied mechanically or in a legalistic fashion is driven home in many of our classical texts. This is aptly illustrated by a *sloka,* which translates as…

> A *vaidya* who comprehends the principles of *rasa,* etc., would discard a textually prescribed treatment if not wholesome to the patient in a given situation; on the contrary, he would adopt treatments that are helpful to the patient, even if they do not find a mention in the texts.

In conclusion, one could sum up some aspects of the traditional Indian systems of knowledge, specifically theory construction and its relation to popular knowledge. The main feature is that the theories do not employ a great degree of 'formalisation' in the sense of providing laws or rules that are 'absolute' and can be blindly applied outside of or irrespective of the context of their formulation. The terms and variables used in the theory and laws are closely related to actual observed phenomena or measured quantities. This does not mean that the theories lack rigour, precision or power. Thus the laws, theories and their terminology have an active and intimate relation to the popular mode of discourse on the subject and the 'folk knowledge' relating to it.

This points to a very important feature of our science and technology, which is that its knowledge, theories and principles are not meant to be reposed in a small number of experts, institutions or texts, but are created and shared on a wide scale by even ordinary folk, who are the day-to-day practitioners of the arts and sciences. In fact, though we have used, for want of a better term, 'folk knowledge' to denote knowledge that lies with our people, its connotation is quite different from the modern context.

In the modern, Western view, 'folklore' is used to denote relatively unreliable knowledge that prevails with the common people. On the other hand, classical or 'proper' scientific knowledge uses its own methods, terminology, theories and abstractions and resides in a different body of people, namely the experts. But in our tradition, this kind of sharp, qualitative difference does not seem to exist.

Folk practitioners are also equally the innovators in the frontiers of their discipline and the theories and technical categories belong to their domain as well. If we consider a highly developed branch of Indian science such as medicine, the basic theories at its foundation, such as the *Panchabhuta* theory of matter and the *Tridosa* theory of causation of disease and its treatment, we discover that they are a part of the common knowledge of even the tribal people. A number of technical terms such as *vata, pitta, kapha, agni, rasa, usna, sita and virya* are all part of the household vocabulary.

The expert seems to play a very different kind of role here, namely that of systematising the corpus of commonly held knowledge. For example, in a discussion about the role of the grammarian, the famous grammarian Patanjali says:

> He who has the use of a pot goes to a potter's house and says, 'Make a pot; I have to use it'. But no one similarly goes to the house of a grammarian and says, 'Coin words; I shall make use of them'.

Thus there is no looking down upon common folk or lay practitioners; on the contrary, the *sastras* repeatedly assert that it is in the concrete particular and its use in real situations that the truth of the *sastras* ultimately resides. The traditional view about the value of knowledge that prevails with the people in general can be seen from the following *sloka*, wherein Caraka advises the *vaidyas*: "By building upon the primary knowledge of cowherds, *tapasvis*, those who dwell in forest, hunters, the uses, names and form of plants, *sàstric* principles can be applied to discover their biological properties."[35]

---

[35] *Caraka Samhita* edited by P. V. Sharma (1983). Varanasi: Chowkhambha Orientalia, *Sutrasthana,* Chapter 1, verse: 120-22.

Western scholars, however, do not accept anything as proper theory unless it is expressed in the Western cultural mould. For over two thousand years, India has been the manufacturer of the famous 'Wootz Steel', which was much sought after and exported to the Middle East and the Roman Empire for centuries. Not only was Wootz stronger than other known forms of steel, but also the conversion of iron ore to steel was faster through the Indian process than by the known European methods. In a letter to the Royal Asiatic Society of Great Britain and Ireland in 1837, J.M. Heath observed:[36]

> Iron is converted into cast steel by the natives of India in two hours and half, with an application of heat that in this country (i.e., England) would be considered quite inadequate to produce such an effect; while at Sheffield it requires at least four hours to melt blistered steel in wind furnaces of the best construction, although the crucibles in which the steel is melted are at a white heat when the metal is put into them, and in the Indian process the crucibles are put into the furnace quite cold.

But he also assures the readers: "... The Indian steel maker of course knows nothing of the theory of his operations. Experience may have taught him that he can make iron pass into steel ..." Heath felt that it was impossible "that the process was discovered by any scientific induction." One can quote dozens of examples where the 'charge' against indigenous Indian science or technology is not that it lacks rigour or precision, or that it does not work, but only that it is not proper science in the modern, western sense of the term.

It is now generally acknowledged that we have a highly developed, indigenous knowledge system of folk and codified streams. It has, however, been organised in a way that is very different from that of modern, Western knowledge. The much-maligned ordinary people of India seem to be as much the innovators as they are repositories of this knowledge. In India, we do not have to take science to the people by any special movement. Traditional

[36] 'On Indian Iron and Steel' by J. M. Heath. Quoted in D. Mushet: *Experiments on Wootz or Indian Steel*. British Museum: 727.k3.

Indian science has its roots in the practices of ordinary people and historically there has been a symbiotic link between folk and classical knowledge. Such an understanding will give us an idea of the manner in which our society organised its knowledge in the past, and also of the larger social principles that have inspired and guided the organisation of our society itself.

5

Contemporary History

Darshan Shankar

Until the beginning of the twentieth century, the transmission of classical medical knowledge was mostly non-institutional, passed on from physician teachers to their chosen students. Historically, there are limited examples of institutionalised medical education; however, towards the end of the colonial period, teaching colleges for traditional medicine had been established. Today, there are about 300 (poorly funded) medical colleges imparting education in various Indian systems of medicine through a five-and-a-half year course, which is similar in structure to Western biomedicine courses. Only a graduate of a recognised medical school is legally entitled to practise traditional medicine.

Although institutionalisation was intended to improve the quality of medical education, this has not happened. While access to education has improved, the quality of education is believed to have deteriorated. An unbroken tradition of more than 3,000 years is thus declining. The dynamism of the Ayurvedic tradition can be inferred from the fact that serious treatises on Ayurveda in the form of aphorisms, compendiums, texts on pharmacy and specialised fields of medicine and surgery, as well as lexicons that were produced between 1500 BC and 1900 AD. In the last 100 years or so, however, there has been a 'lull' in its creativity.

History of Policymaking in Indigenous Medicine

It can be seen from historical records that the European response to indigenous science falls into two phases. The earlier phase was a part of the European quest for useful knowledge from the non-European world. This phase occurred in the seventeenth and early eighteenth centuries, a period corresponding to the time when Europe's interest in India was only trade-related. During this period, the Europeans were curious about the methodology and deeply appreciative of the efficacy of ISM.

One area where indigenous practise produced outstanding results was in smallpox inoculations (see Chapter 4). Another example of outstanding medical practises is in the field of surgery. According to an account by Colonel Kyd:

> In surgery, in which (the Indians) are considered least advanced, they often succeed in removing ulcers and cutaneous eruptions of the worst kinds, including those which have baffled the skills of our surgeons, by the process of inducing inflammation and by means directly opposite to ours and which they have probably long been in obsession of.

Dr H. Scott (MD), in a communication to Sir Joseph Banks, President of the Royal Society, London, wrote:

> The effects of surgical operation are more obvious. They practise with great success the operation of depressing the crystalline lens when it becomes opaque (*sic*) and from time immemorial they have cut for the stone at the same place, which they now do in Europe. These are curious facts and I believe unknown to us.

But perhaps it is in the area of plastic surgery that the Indian tradition was greatly advanced from early times. This had an impact on the practise of the art all over the world. As S.C. Almast once wrote: "Twice did this art spread from India to the rest of the world."[37]

The knowledge of rhinoplastic procedures was probably transferred to Western civilisation by the free interchange of thought and experience between Hindu, Arab, Persian, Greek, Nestorian and Jewish scholars. Celsus, the Roman who lived from 25 BC to 50 AD, was probably the earliest West European to describe the Indian methods of plastic operations on the nose. The *Susruta Samhita* was mentioned as *Kitabe Sushrud* by Ibn Abi 'Usaybia' (1203–1269 AD), the first historian of Arabian medicine. It is said that during the reign of Al Mansur (died 775 AD), an Indian medical work

[37] These and other examples can be found in *Indian Science and Technology in the Eighteenth Century* by Dharmapal (1971). Hyderabad: Academy of Gandhian Studies.

by Susruta was rendered into Arabic by Manke, the Hindu court physician, at the suggestion of Wazie Yahyaibn Khalid. The practical secrets of rhinoplastic operations spread from India through Arabia and Persia to Egypt, from where it entered Italy. In Sicily during the fifteenth century, Branca used cheek grafts to reconstruct the proud noses of hot-blooded swordsmen. His son Antonio tried grafts from the arm and by the late sixteenth century, Tagliacozzi had published his work on the Italian method of arm flap rhinoplasty.[38]

Despite such accounts of competence, indigenous surgery, like smallpox vaccination, was legally prohibited during the first half of British rule. This was part of a deliberate strategy by the British to undermine the self-reliance of Indians. By mid-nineteenth century, Allopathy had become the sole recipient of state patronage, leading to a decline of the indigenous systems. Surgery became dysfunctional and several traditional institutions of learning were forced to close down. Not surprisingly, this had an adverse impact on the morale of traditional practitioners. It is common for a section of historians and scientists to explain this decline as a natural process by which a traditional body of knowledge loses its relevance in the face of the superior rationality of modern science. Here, however, it is clear that the decline can be directly pegged to a political process that favoured the Western system of medicine and Western knowledge in general — to the detriment of indigenous systems.

The pre-Independence movement attempted to restore an Indian 'identity', but taking place as it did when indigenous social, political and economic institutions and traditions were being rapidly replaced by Western models, it was inevitably influenced by Western ideas and social forms. This influence is evident in the content of the ideological debate that emerged during this century on the question of how to revitalise Ayurveda. The revivalist movement led by the Indian National Congress developed two ideological streams. The first held that indigenous medicine should be taught and practised in its classical or *suddh* form, while the second, which was directly influenced by Western ideas, held that Western science needed to be integrated into indigenous theory, principles and practice in order to make it more complete. Liberal social circles saw the first position as retrograde and orthodox, although they had made

[38] *Homo Faber* by Claude Alvares (1984). New Delhi: Mentor Publications.

no systematic assessment of the epistemological issues involved or the competence of indigenous systems to deal with contemporary health care needs. They were more impressed by the easily demonstrated experimental methods and technology associated with Western medical science, as also its superior value in the job market. The social organisation of indigenous medicine during this period also began to alter. There was the birth of a new work culture, aptly described by the term 'professionalisation'. This professional culture resulted in several significant changes in the functioning of traditional systems.

- Formal colleges of Indian medicine were created with a time-bound syllabus, an examination system and an impersonal teaching methodology. This replaced the traditional family-based, *guru–sisya* relationship. The latter had its own time-tested culture of learning and unique pedagogic principles, i.e., *adhiti* — memorise, *bodham* — analyse, *acaranam* – – practise, and *pracaranam* — teach.
- Dispensaries and hospitals similar in design to Allopathic inpatient and outpatient departments were established in order to provide health services.
- Pharmacies were set up for the small-scale production and marketing of medicines.
- Professional associations, a board for the registration of medical practitioners, and medical journals were initiated.

Correspondingly, the traditional physician, too, gradually moved into a clinic to prescribe commercially manufactured drugs, switching over to a disease-oriented practice and hospital-centred care. All aspects of this new 'professional' culture from the West were accepted uncritically and without much debate.

In 1920, the Indian National Congress passed its first resolution in Nagpur, whereby indigenous medicine received political support for the first time after a hundred years of being ignored by colonial policies. Representative provincial governments set up special committees to define the necessary steps to be taken. The Government of India, under the chairmanship of R.N. Chopra, also set up a Central Committee in 1946 for the purpose.

The basic recommendation of the Chopra Committee Report (1948)[39] was for the integration of traditional and Western systems of medicine, which was translated into a blueprint for a national health plan: 'We have come to the conclusion that such a synthesis, though not easy and (definitely) time-consuming, is not only possible but practicable and essential.' The committee also compared the syllabi of the two systems (see Table 5.1):

Table 5.1

Ayurveda and Western Medicine — Differences in Syllabi

Ayurveda Section	Western Section
1 *Padartha vijnana* (*darsanas*) (Physics and chemistry pertaining to Ayurveda)	1 Basic sciences (biology)
2 *Sarira*	2 Anatomy
3 *Dosa-dhatu mala vijnana*	3 Physiology
4 *Dravya guna vijnana, rasa sastra* and *ausadha nirmana*	4 Materia medica
5 *Svastha vrtta*	5 Hygiene and public health
6 *Nidana* (*roga-vijnana*)	6 Pathology
7 *Kaya cikitsa*	7 General medicine
8 *Salya* and *salakya*	8 Surgery, including diseases of the eye, ear nose and throat
9 *Prasuti-tantra*, *stri-roga*, *kaumarabhrtya*	9 Midwifery, gynaecology and paediatrics
10 *Agada-tantra* and *vyavahara-ayurveda*	10 Toxicology and medical jurisprudence

[39] Chopra Committee Report, 1948. See also 'Indigenous Health Services' by D. Shankar (1992) in *State of India's Health* edited by A. Mukhopadhyay. New Delhi: Voluntary Health Association of India.

The report stated:

> It is to be noted that, although similar subjects have been included in both sections, the teaching of some of these is not being done in a correlated manner. We, however, hold that the study should as far as possible be made more 'synthetic and comparative' rather than as a detached study of pure Allopathic principles and practices. For this purpose the teaching of Ayurvedic and Western subjects should preferably be by teachers holding an allopathic degree as well as a diploma or degree in Indian medicine. In this way, in the course of time, the lecture notes in each subject could form the basis for the preparation of what may be called 'unified textbooks' suitable for use by every student of medicine in India, no matter what the special branch—Allopathy, Ayurveda, Siddha or Unani.

The recommendations of the Chopra Committee were rejected. In retrospect, it is clear that the committee's concept of integration was wholly ignorant of the epistemological considerations involved in a synthesis of Western biomedicine and Ayurveda.

Despite political support in the pre-Independence period, the ISM community remained deeply divided on ideological grounds regarding its relationship with Western medicine. The divide, however, should not be seen as a squabble between orthodox and progressive forces (which is the common view), but as a foundational debate, which has its roots in epistemology.

This revivalist movement at the dawn of pre-Independence, however, left untouched the revitalisation of the *lok svasthya paramparas* or folk medicine and chose to concentrate on the *sastriya* (codified) stream alone.

Recommendations of official committees

***Bhore committee (1944-46)*:** The sovereign Government of India in effect accepted the Bhore Committee's blueprint for national health services after independence. This was based entirely on the Allopathic system of medicine. The rather disgraceful recommendation of the committee regarding the future of ISM was to "create a chair for the study of history of medicine in the

All India Institute of Medical Sciences, New Delhi, wherein the indigenous systems should be studied as part of medical history." Fortunately, this recommendation was not accepted.

***Chopra committee (1948)*:** The alternative blueprint suggested by the Chopra Committee gave ISM an equal role in rural and urban services. However, the Government of India rejected this report as well.

***C.G. Pant committee (1950)*:** The Pant Committee was appointed to follow up the major recommendations made by the Chopra Committee. It rejected the idea of a common, integrated syllabus for all medical colleges (including Allopathy) and suggested instead that research be initiated on indigenous systems in order to establish their validity. In 1956, a Central Institute of Research was created for this purpose in Jamnagar, Gujarat.

***Dave committee (1954)*:** The Dave Committee prepared a model, integrated syllabus only for ISM teaching colleges that combined indigenous and modern sciences. It also recommended the same privileges for registered medical practitioners of ISM as for Allopathic practitioners. ISM colleges functioned on this integrated syllabus till 1962.

Mudaliar committee (1961): This committee recommended the return of ISM to their *suddh* or purely classical form. It thus did away with integrated courses, which were abandoned by 1962.

Udupa committee (1968): The Udupa Committee recommended the gradual integration of modern medicine into ISM, the establishment of three postgraduate institutes, a research council for ISM, and an independent council for the regulation of educational standards in ISM.

Financing Health Services

During the Seventh, Eighth and Ninth Plan periods, ISM (including Homeopathy, Naturopathy and Yoga) received around 3 per cent of the national health budget. State allocations varied, with only the government of Kerala allocating 13 per cent of its medical budget for ISM. Bengal allocated less than 0.5 per cent. In general, ISM are better supported in Kerala, Tamil Nadu, Karnataka, Maharashtra, Gujarat and Rajasthan and less so in northern states like Madhya Pradesh, Himachal Pradesh, Uttar Pradesh, Punjab and Haryana. The West Bengal and Bihar state governments remain unresponsive to them.

Box 5.1

Developments in ISM Research (1960–1991)

Role of ICMR

The Indian Council of Medical Research (ICMR) was a pioneer in the pharmacological and clinical evaluation of ISM drugs. It was the sole body responsible for the work done between 1960 and 1970. Its efforts have been largely directed at validating ISM drugs along modern parameters.

In 1969-70, the ICMR was divested of this central role in directing research programmes on ISM and the responsibility was entrusted to a specially-created autonomous body — the Central Council for Research in Indian Medicine (Ayurveda, Unani, Siddha) and Homeopathy (CCRIMH). Since 1970, this body has been the central research agency for ISM. However, the ICMR continues to undertake clinical research on traditional medicine though it is no longer the nodal agency. Even after 30 years of research in ISM, the ICMR has not come out with any comprehensive publication that can advise Indian medical professionals on how and what aspects of ISM can be integrated with mainstream Indian medical practice.

In 1978, the CCRIMH was divided into four independent councils for conducting research in different spheres of indigenous medicine:

1 Central Council for Research in Ayurveda and Siddha (CCRAS)
2 Central Council for Research in Unani Medicine (CCRUM)
3 Central Council for Research in Homeopathy (CCRH)
4 Central Council for Research in Naturopathy and Yoga (CCRNY)

Today, the CCRAS has 90 centres — small and medium — engaged in various research activities all over the country. The CCRUM has an additional 29 centres engaged in research.

ISM Health Extension Services (1947-2001)

ISM health delivery services in rural and urban areas are not in any way linked to the national primary health care services. While they are effective and popular in some states like Kerala and Tamil Nadu, in other states their impact is negligible. Around 23,000 Ayurvedic, Unani, and Siddha dispensaries, fully funded by state governments, are operational in various parts of the country. They function without any orientation to national health goals, and there has been no review in post-independent India of how to make the ISM health services sector more effective. Twenty-two states even have directorates for ISM health services, but these function parallel to and are independent of the State Directorate of Health Services, which manages primary health care programmes.

Table 5.2 describes the structure of indigenous systems of medicine, as they exist today.

Table 5.2

Indigenous Systems of Medicine

1 Grassroots level in village communities all over India	7 lakh midwives.[40] 60,000 village bonesetters 60,000 herbal medicare healers (excluding spiritual healers), including those who specialise in areas like *marma* (acupressure), *netra*, *danta cikitsa*, paralytic conditions, mental diseases, *visa* (poisons), *pasu cikitsa* (veterinary) Millions of housewives with knowledge of home	These folk healers constitute the *lok svasthya paramparas* or traditions. They are decentralised, autonomous and self-reliant with regional variations and are supported entirely by village communities They use local resources. 8000 species of medicinal plants are used in *lok svasthya paramparas* all over India, apart from

(contd.)

[40] These are rough estimates. Seven lakh corresponds to roughly one midwife in each village and 60,000 covers approximately 10 per cent of India's villages. There is a need to carry out an all-India census of *lok svasthya paramparas* along the lines of the special census on artisans carried out in 1961.

(Table 5.2 contd.)

	remedies, therapeutic diets, promotive herbs and indigenous nutrition principles and practices	minerals and animal products
2 Non-government ISM centres	Small clinics of excellence (*sastriya*) dealing with bone setting, treatment of polio, treatment of eye diseases, arthritis, skin diseases, dental care, *acupressure*, *panca karma*, mental diseases, *ausadhikarana*, cardiac diseases, paediatrics, *visa* and mother-and-child care exist in various parts of the country. Some of these clinics have facilities for a small number of in-patients. Whereas some of them function on a commercial scale (like private Allopathy centres), most of them are accessible to the common folk	In some of the traditional centres outstanding work is being carried out which can contribute to world medicine; for example, in a hospital for polio patients in Coimbatore, a respected, modern, orthopaedic surgeon reported that patients were cured of the clubfoot deformity with the use of herbal oils for softening bony tissues Similarly, wasted muscles have gained 'inches' in dimension (girth) by massaging with special oils. In Rajkot, Gujarat, as also in Pune in Maharashtra, there are traditional dentists who conduct painless extractions using a yogic technique for anaesthetising the patient In Kerala, there is a *netra* clinic where the

(contd.)

(Table 5.2 contd.)

		development of cataract is arrested in the early stages with the use of Ayurvedic medicines
		In Cannanore, snakebites caused by the Russell's viper are treated with Ayurvedic drugs. Modern doctors work along with traditional physicians at this centre. Modern doctors report that the diagnostics of snakebites in Ayurvedic texts is very elaborate and far more refined than in other medical systems
		Effective treatment for arthritis can be found in Indian systems of medicine and there are several competent centres engaged in this work. The Arya Vaidya Chikitsalayam in Coimbatore and the Kottakkal Hospitals treat hundreds of patients from the world over every year
		Several centres treat diseases of the gastro-intestinal tract, respiratory diseases and chronic skin conditions

(contd.)

(Table 5.2 contd.)

3 Official ISM institutions set up by the Government of India and state governments	300 undergraduate teaching colleges, seven postgraduate centres Central Research Councils for Ayurveda and Siddha (90 units) and Unani (29 units) Network of dispensaries, mostly in rural areas, delinked from mainstream primary health care services (supported by state governments) Thirteen state-run pharmacies, 'small-scale' production units have been set up in various states. Their production is used exclusively for supply to state-run health services in ISM	Qualitatively, the output of official institutions, teaching, research and services is poor. This is generally true for all government sector activities as compared to the private or voluntary sector Compared to official support for Allopathic teaching, research and service institutions, it should be noted that ISM receive less than 3% of the national health budget
4 Private sector in ISM	Individual private practitioners form the bulk of the private sector. At the end of 2001, according to statistics issued by the Ministry of Health and Family Welfare, there were almost 500,000 *Ayurvedic*, *Unani* and *Siddha* registered practitioners in the	While there is a growing trend to emulate the commercial style of Allopathic medical practice in urban areas, on the whole the private sector in ISM has not become completely commercialised. In recent years, some multinational

(contd.)

(Table 5.2 contd.)

	country. There are very few private hospitals. The largest investment of the private sector in ISM is in pharmaceuticals. According to the Planning and Evaluation Cell of the Ministry of Health and Family Welfare, in 2001 there were about 9,300 licensed pharmacies. The majority (around 6,000) have a turnover of less than one crore; only 10% report turnovers of over 50 crore Despite the growing size of the pharmaceutical industry, it has not been governed by any rigorous quality control or pharmaceutical standards. However, GOI has recently introduced a GMP code to be applicable from June 2002	companies have also entered the market with Ayurvedic products This may be seen as a purely commercial decision because ISM drugs are exempted from excise
5 Professional associations of ISM practitioners	The oldest association is the Ayurvedic Congress established in 1907. It supports the *suddh* form of Ayurveda and is reported to have a large membership and several state branches	Although bodies like the All India Ayurvedic Congress and the Unani physicians under the leadership of Hakim Ajmal Khan played a leading role in the pre-Independence survival movement, in

(contd.)

(Table 5.2 contd.)

	A national association of medical professionals who believe in integrating ISM with the allopathic system also exists. Most of the members are practitioners of indigenous medicine In Tamil Nadu, Siddha practitioners have active associations which lobby effectively with the state government In Ladakh and Spiti there are associations of *Amchis*, who practice medicine based on the *gso-rig-pa* tradition There are a few (though not very active) associations of Unani practitioners	the post-independence period their role has been rather limited. The professional associations have failed to work out a larger vision of what contributions ISM can make to national health goals

Although ISM research councils lay claim to several achievements, in reality none of their findings has actually penetrated mainstream medical practice. The orthodox traditional physicians reject the findings on the grounds that 'single drug, single disease' is not an ISM proposition at all. Therefore, any findings related to any disease that advocates the use of a single drug are considered necessarily incomplete. The Allopaths have also rejected such findings, as they believe that the clinical research has been conducted without the rigour that is demanded for universal acceptance.

Where Does the Future Lie?

The ideology of Swadeshi in the pre- and post-Independence periods has ensured a permanent place for indigenous systems of medicine in Indian society. It has rescued them from ignominy and restored a certain measure of dignity and patronage that was completely absent during colonial rule. Despite this, ISM has not flourished in independent India. There appear to be two reasons for this: first, the Indian Allopathic community supported by health policymakers has continued to play the colonial role in discrediting ISM; and second, the ISM community itself has remained inert. It has not risen to the contemporary challenge of health care despite the existence of a favourable political climate. In very recent times, there has been a shift in perception and a new 'openness' to collaboration. This openness is due to the global shift in health care policies wherein the complementary and alternative medicine (CAM) movement is gaining new public space.

The ISM has allowed them to be discredited through their acceptance of wrongly designed research schemes. Research designs for ISM in post-Independence India have been based on the assumption that the science of these systems can be validated 'only' through modern, Allopathic medical parameters. In the first place, the correlation of diseases and symptoms recognised by Allopathy with those described by ISM is not well established. Second, unlike Allopathy, the indigenous systems do not advocate one drug for one disease. This is because their theory of cause and effect is based on a 'systemic diagnosis' wherein a particular disease may manifest itself differently in different groups of people. From the ISM point of view, therefore, it is 'unscientific' to look for a single-drug therapy. Third, the theory of drug action in ISM is explained in terms of the ability of the drug to restore homeostasis. In Allopathy, on the other hand, drug action is generally explained in terms of its antibiotic activity. Despite such differences, clinical and drug research in post-independent India has attempted to assess ISM along the lines of modern systems. No wonder, then, that research carried out by the Indian Council for Medical Research (ICMR), Central Council for Research in Ayurveda and Siddha (CCRAS) and other ISM centres over the past 25 years has yielded indifferent results.

The ISM community still has not recovered from the condemnation it has faced over the last 200 years. It could have promoted an innovative scheme of intercultural research to establish its ability to manage various diseases using indigenous diagnostic, pharmacological and therapeutic logic. Having proved its success through well documented case studies, it could have stood its ground, insisting that the reasons for the success of ISM could only be understood if interested professionals were prepared to study the basic principles and diagnostics of the indigenous health sciences instead of seeking to understand ISM through superficial correlations between the concepts of ISM and Allopathy. However, even the favourable climate in post-independent India could not help the ISM community recover its nerve. It uncritically accepted the research designs imposed by Allopaths in the hope that the clinical principles of classical texts would somehow be validated. This was a compromise that helped only in stunting the development of the indigenous systems. It has also led to the disorientation of teaching programmes. The adoption of the integrated syllabus until 1962 — which was more a mixture than a creative synthesis — and of the formal, institution-based teaching methods destroyed the traditional system of teaching. While there has been a huge expansion in ISM teaching institutions, the expansion can be attributed more to market pressures to create more professional courses than to the revival of ISM.

However, there are some hopeful signs. Creative and outstanding work is being done in small, non-government institutions and clinics in different parts of the country. The best ISM physicians and institutions are in the non-governmental sector.

The most functional and largest health delivery service sector of ISM is the 'people's health system'. This is the decentralised, community-managed, folk medicine system which functions at the grassroots and delivers far more than all the official primary health care institutions. However, this health culture is ignored in health policy. Further, the *lok svasthya paramparas* are not without weaknesses. The task of revitalising the local traditions, confirming what is sound, adding to what is incomplete, and removing what is distorted is the greatest challenge for the primary health care movement in India, because the *lok svasthya paramparas* represent the only sustainable, self-reliant forms of health care for village India.

Indigenous health sciences and their widespread folk traditions are our cultural heritage. The revitalisation of traditional medicine is not the responsibility of the traditional practitioners alone, but of the nation as a whole. A genuinely modern India will emerge only when the present generation of Indian scientists frees itself from the prejudices that have turned 'tradition and modern' into mutually exclusive categories. Only when Indian Allopathic medical practitioners work together with respect and with regard for whatever is of contemporary relevance in our heritage, will we have what could be called a truly modern 'Indian' system of health care.

Bibliography

Mukhopadhyay, A. (1991) *Report on State of India's Health*. New Delhi: Voluntary Health Association of India.

Poleman, H. J. and P. G. Roche (1939) Aspects of Caesarean Section in India. *Journal of American Oriental Society*, pp.17–21.

Wise, T. A. (1860) *Commentary on the Hindu System of Medicine*. London: Trubner and Co.

SECTION II

Accounts of Living Health Traditions

6

Documenting and Revitalising Local Health Traditions

A. Hafeel, T.S. Suma and P.M. Unnikrishnan

In this chapter we describe a programme that represents a first step toward the renewal of medicinal plant cultivation in households, and also perhaps a first step in the direction of health security. The programme eventually included 60,000 households in rural Tamil Nadu, a state in southern India. It involved the training of several volunteer groups and women's organisations spread throughout the state.

The response was swift and encouraging. The women volunteers themselves ensured a 'multiplication effect' by bringing many others from the village into the programme. These people came of their own accord and were even willing to contribute large sums of money — which is especially commendable, as the programme had targeted the rural poor. It ended the misconception that programmes for the poor can only be carried out in a spirit of charity; on the contrary, we found that people, however poor, were willing to pay, provided we clearly explained the benefits to them and won their trust.

The chapters in the first section of this book focused on providing a theoretical overview. In this section, we will try and give the readers a 'feel' of large-scale community work. The current and next chapter follow the implementation of a large project involving an entire community, tracking it all the way from the most preliminary groundwork and estimates towards its final (yet renewable and replicable) end.

Documentation of Local Health Traditions

Local health traditions (LHTs) or community and habitat-specific practises, beliefs and customs related to health, form an integral part of the local lifestyle and include all aspects of health care like prevention, cure and promotion. Home remedies and health-related customs that are prevalent in millions of households are living expressions of these traditions. These diverse and informal systems are passed on from generation to generation by word of mouth through millions of ordinary households as well as by specialised folk healers.

By specialised folk healers we mean practitioners like bonesetters, poisonous bite healers, traditional birth attendants (TBAs) and folk veterinary healers who comprise the service providers of this health care system. Specialised skills in these areas include, among others, diagnostic methods such as *nadi pariksa* (pulse examination), *mutra pariksa* (examination of urine), *visa pariksa* (diagnostic and prognostic methods used in cases of poisoning), and *varma kalai* (diagnosis and treatment using vital points in the body). Diagnosis and reduction techniques for fractures, emergency care like treating natural poisons, specialised eye care, and treatment of individual, organ-related conditions are some of the other skills of traditional healers.

In India, they exist throughout the country, parallel to the codified, indigenous systems of medicine such as Ayurveda, Siddha, Western biomedicine and Homeopathy, and are dependent on local natural resources. It may surprise readers to know that there are about 8,000 plant species and more than 200 animal and mineral sources being used by 4,639 ethnic Indian communities.[41] This and the following chapter examine in detail how LHTs can be studied and promoted.

These time-tested health traditions still serve a vast majority of India's rural population. According to a Voluntary Health Association of India report, only 6.3 per cent of rural deliveries are institutionalised; the rest are managed birth attendants who are either trained by the government or have received training in their own local health tradition.[42]

The recent increase in the demand for natural products has encouraged the emergence of commercial interest in the resources used by LHTs, which

[41] All India Coordinated Research Project on Ethnobiology, Final Technical Report Phase 1 (1987-1990), Regional Research Institute, Central Council for Research in Ayurveda and Siddha, Government of India, Kerala.

[42] 'Health Systems and Services' in *State of India's Health* edited by A. Mukhopadhyay (1992). New Delhi: Voluntary Health Association of India.

are now tapped by national and international pharmaceutical companies for drug development. A recently developed drug for hepatitis from the plant *Phyllanthus amarus* is based on the knowledge of the natives of southern India; the product *Jivani*, based on the plant (*Trichopus zeylanicus)*, is used as an immuno-modulator, and *Piper longum* (piperine) is used as a bio-availability enhancer. These are but a few examples of drugs patented from the traditional knowledge base; there are many more such potential candidates awaiting patents.

However, despite the promise of self-reliance in the health care sector, the present political and social attitude towards LHTs is discouraging. It is observed that these traditions are being eroded at an alarming pace. As has been noted in an earlier chapter, the practitioners' lack of self-confidence and their marginalisation by the politically dominant medical systems are major contributors to this erosion.

The present Western medicine-based health care system in India is highly capital-intensive and technocentric, and hence dependent on external resources. Its coverage of rural households is estimated to be around 30 per cent of the population (national level), with the percentage being as low as 3 per cent in certain areas.[43] This situation demands a movement that incorporates local resources and local knowledge for effective practises in the health care system. The process of understanding LHTs and locating effective practises in the rich, local medical cultures has not yet gained momentum. Researching effective practises through elaborate pharmacological and clinical trials is a colossal task. Validating a single practice would involve five to eight years of laboratory research with a huge amount of capital investment.

Because of this situation, the Foundation for Revitalisation of Local Health Traditions (FRLHT) set about attempting a transformation. The task that FRLHT set itself for 1998–2000 was to develop a methodology for documentation and participatory assessment in order to promote positively assessed local health measures. The objective was to come up with a methodology that would identify effective community health practices at the

---

[43] Ibid.

household level through a participatory process. This 'Rapid Assessment of Local Health Traditions (RALHT)' approach, as it was called, involves a judicious blend of local experiences as well as the clinical experiences of other Indian health care systems and Indian medical literature such as Ayurveda, Siddha and Unani. We explicate here the steps involved in the RALHT process, as well as the results obtained.

This project on comprehensive documentation and rapid assessment of local health traditions was carried out in two distinct phases. The initial phase included the collection of data from households and folk healers. A cursory description is given in this chapter of the status and diversity of health practises throughout the southern and eastern parts of the country. The second phase consisted of participatory approaches in finding priority health conditions and assessing effective remedies for them (see Chapter 7 for details on the second phase).

Development of Data Collection Tools

Comprehensive documentation

Questionnaires were developed to record resources, knowledge, and the socio–cultural aspects of health traditions from households and healers. Different subsets of questionnaires were designed in order to record different levels of knowledge and practise. Initially, two separate sets of household questionnaires on home remedies and food regimens were devised. Following this, five subsets of questionnaires were distributed to field assistants for documentation. These were:

- *Mrga vaidyas* (veterinary practitioners),
- *Visa vaidyas* (poison specialists),
- Traditional Birth Attendants (midwives),
- Traditional Bonesetters,
- General (those who treat general/specific organ/system-related health conditions).

Prior to the documentation phase, a pilot study was carried out in four different field locations of Kerala, Tamil Nadu, Maharashtra and Karnataka,

Figure 6.1
Field Collaborators
Project on Revitalisation of Local Health Traditions

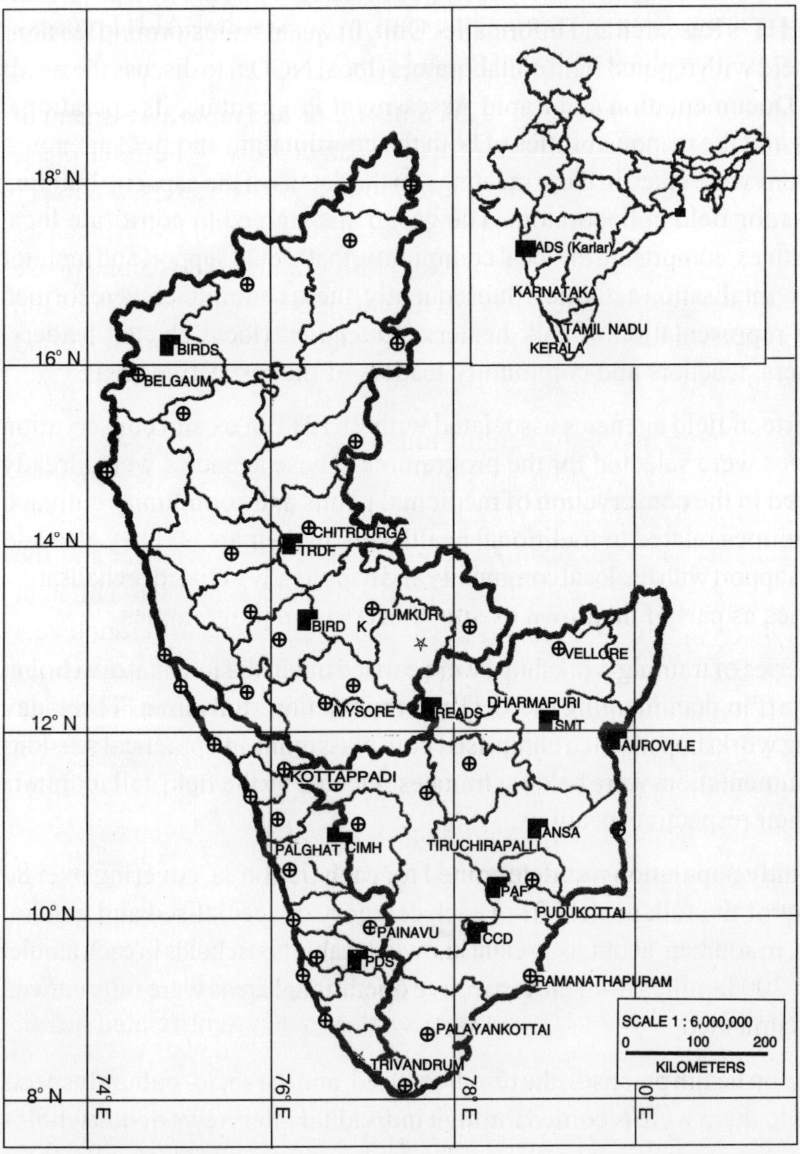

Foundation for Revitalisation of Local Health Traditions, Bangalore, India

which served as a base for designing the questionnaires and finalising the documentation approach for the study (see Figure 6.1 for locations). Data on the folk healer population was also collected.

Before launching the study, which was coordinated by the ISM physicians of FRLHT's Research and Informatics Unit, frequent brainstorming sessions were held with reputed field collaborators (local NGOs) to discuss the needs of the Documentation and Rapid Assessment Programme, its operational details and the responsibilities of both the coordinating and field agencies. Decisions were taken in these meetings on the details of the capacity building process for field collaborators. The group also agreed to constitute local committees, comprising the local community, that would support and monitor all the revitalisation activities. Subsequently, these committees were formed with a representation of folk healers, *panchayat* (local elected leaders) members, teachers and community leaders of the respective areas.

Thirteen field agencies associated with FRLHT in ex situ conservation activities were selected for the programme. These agencies were already involved in the conservation of medicinal plants and community outreach programmes related to traditional health care in their areas. They also had a good rapport with the local community and had already initiated revitalisation activities as part of their own ex situ conservation programmes.

A series of training workshops were carried out in the four states to orient field staff in documenting the LHTs in their action study area. Three-day training workshops, which comprised both classroom and practical sessions on documentation, were held for trainees selected by the field collaborators from their respective localities.

A study population was determined for each field area, covering over 80 per cent of the folk healers from each category of specialised and general healers. In addition, about six to eight knowledgeable households in each hamlet of 100–200 families from the respective operational areas were interviewed and documented.

Data on health practises, the resources used, and the socio–cultural aspects related to them were recorded through individual interviews of households and folk healers and verified by the field-level coordinators. Data obtained from the field was then translated from the respective vernacular to specific programmable formats in English. Some of the general findings of the study are given below:

Ethnography

India has a high ethnic diversity of over 4,000 communities. During the course of this study, the field teams interacted with informants from 190 ethnic communities. Even in this small study sample, the variety in practise, knowledge and resources was extraordinary. The vast knowledge of traditional healing often consists of different specialisations. For example, the *Kuruba* community is involved in cattle rearing and most of the *Mrga vaidyas* (veterinarians) are from this community. The *Ambatta* women have traditionally served as birth attendants. The *Vannans*, whose usual occupation is to wash clothes, are traditionally known for treating children's diseases.[44]

At the household level, home remedies, food and nutritional aspects and health related customs vary by geographical region, religion and community. These are alive in the form of various health practises of different communities and relate to their mental, physical and social well-being. The depth of knowledge differs from community to community and, of course, as we shall see in the section on household traditions, their level of knowledge about remedies and food is different from that of the healers.

An important factor in ethnographic considerations is that like many other forms of folk knowledge, health traditions are passed on from generation to generation by word of mouth. The making of a folk healer involves a rigorous process of training under a *guru*, which is the traditional way of transferring skills and understanding. Sessions of practical training and oral teachings from the *guru* span a number of years. Intensive and practical, the training includes such areas as the identification of medicines, diagnosis of health problems, prescription of appropriate medicine, and the preparation of the medicine. It is not rare for prayers and rituals to be associated with this transfer of knowledge.

---

[44] *Castes and Tribes of South India* by E. Thurston and K. Rangachari (1993). Madras: Asian Educational Services.

Healers have certain criteria for recruiting students. These include a consideration of the moral standards of the pupils and may involve several days of observation. Criteria that were repeatedly cited during the study are:

- Love and compassion towards the ailing
- Altruism
- Faith in god
- Tolerance
- Willingness to serve the patients at any time
- Not being money-minded or greedy
- An interest in learning and healing.

Sometimes, an added condition was that the disciples be family members or blood relations. Gender was also a consideration, particularly in the case of midwives. Where household health practises are concerned, the elders pass on their knowledge to the younger generation as part of their lifestyle and customs.

Traditionally, healing is considered to be a duty rather than a profession. *Vaidyas* respond to the query: "Why did you decide to take up healing?" with expressions like "Doing service", "It is a family tradition". This is substantiated by the high incidence of healers who are only part-time practitioners. In villages, they provide people with health services irrespective of time, caste, or economic and social barriers.

The feeling that the healer is 'one of us' enhances the community's access to traditional health service providers. Since *vaidyas* understand and are familiar with the patients' personal and societal environment, their approach to healing is holistic.

Food and disease

While considering causes of illnesses related to food, its availability, quality and the eating habits of the patient are considered. Stale food, 'outside food', adulterated food items, vegetables and grains grown using artificial manures and pesticides are regarded as harmful. Further, the addition of artificial agents to beautify and enhance taste is seen as disease causing. Mixing foods of various natures and from different places is also considered to be a factor that causes disease.

Environment and disease

Cold weather, the monsoon season and hot summers are generally regarded as factors that generate or increase disease. For instance, rheumatic disorders, old age health problems like body pain, and chronic asthma increase during the monsoons. In the *Karkidaka* month (monsoon) in Kerala, people are advised to take precautions against *vata*[45] vitiating problems. An example is the *Karkidaka kanji*—a medicinal porridge. Change of weather is related to some respiratory problems and certain fevers. Women working under the hot sun are susceptible to *vetta* or white discharge.

Habits and diseases

Modern lifestyles are also stated to cause illness due to the psychological shift from a relaxed life to a tense and hurried one. 'Bad habits', such as carelessness, lack of personal hygiene, long nails, not having proper and regular baths, improper sleeping and eating habits, smoking and the intake of alcohol are additional factors that invite disease. Greed and harming other individuals and life forms also generate disease.

Some diseases are considered to be genetic — for instance, *Kustham* (a chronic skin condition). Insanity and *Chuzhali*, *Ilakkam* (both regional names for non-specific epilepsy) are also said to be passed on by parents. Maternal eating habits also affect children's health—especially in the context of breastfeeding.

An individual's *prakrti* or constitution also influences susceptibility or immunity to disease. *Sarirabalam, Nalla udampu, Sakti,* etc., are synonyms for a healthy constitution. LHTs use the classical theory of the functional principles—*vata*, *pitha* and *kapha*[46]—and their effect on the state of health (whether balanced or imbalanced) to understand and explain pathogenesis.

---

[45] One among three bodily principles; also known as a disease entity in folk medicine.

[46] These are three functional principles of the body as understood by the classical stream of indigenous medicine. Their balance and imbalance is responsible for health and ill health.

Supernatural powers are also believed to affect the health of an individual. Ill health is often attributed to fate and incurrence of the wrath of the gods. A medical condition called *Amma* in Tamil is believed to occur in individuals who have angered Goddess Kali. According to '*Jataka-Sastram* (a Tamil manuscript on horoscope found in Viruthunagar district of Tamil Nadu), planetary positions, too, have a definite impact on physical and mental health.

A Healthy Life — Local Perspectives

According to the *vaidyas*, the concept of health includes both physical and mental health. The expression *udampum mansum nalla irukkanam* means that both the body and mind should be in good condition. 'Follow the elders style of living and advice, customs and traditions, have nutritious food and live without bad habits' — are some ways by which we can attain good health. Purity of mind, lack of anger, jealousy and greed, and self-control are also ingredients for a healthy life. The spiritual aspect of one's life, as represented by *daiva bhakti* and *samy kumbidal*, is therefore of prime importance.

Folk healers

Folk healers generally fall into some category of specialisation or the other and can therefore manage both human and veterinary systemic health problems as well as emergency care. The management of these conditions needs different techniques, medicinal preparations and resources. Depending on their area of specialisation, the folk healers can be categorised into five groups.

Among the thousand healers who were initially interviewed, the TBAs formed the largest specialised group. They were followed by healers of poisonous bites, traditional veterinary healers and bonesetters, in descending order. A large group of practitioners of different and uncommon specialisation and healers who treat general conditions were put into one general category, which comprised over 50 per cent of the total population interviewed. Among these practitioners, the number of male healers was almost twice that of female healers. The categories of poison healers, bonesetters and veterinary healers were dominated by male *vaidyas*.

Table 6.1

Categories of Healers and Conditions Treated

Speciality	**Treatment given for/ attends to**	**Example**
Visa vaidya	Poisonous bites of animal origin	Treatment for snakebites and scorpion bites
Mrga vaidya	Veterinary conditions	Indigestion, loose motion, foot and mouth, fractures, ulcers, etc.
Traditional bonesetter	Fractures, sprains other injuries related to trauma	Fractures of hands, legs, etc.
Traditional birth attendants (midwives)	Delivery, prenatal and postnatal care	Recipes for the prenatal and postnatal period, normal delivery
General	Organ-related diseases, spiritual healing, paediatrics, gynaecological problems, etc.	Eye diseases, jaundice, gastric problems, headaches, different types of fever, etc.

Figure 6.2 Population of Different Healers (total 1,000)

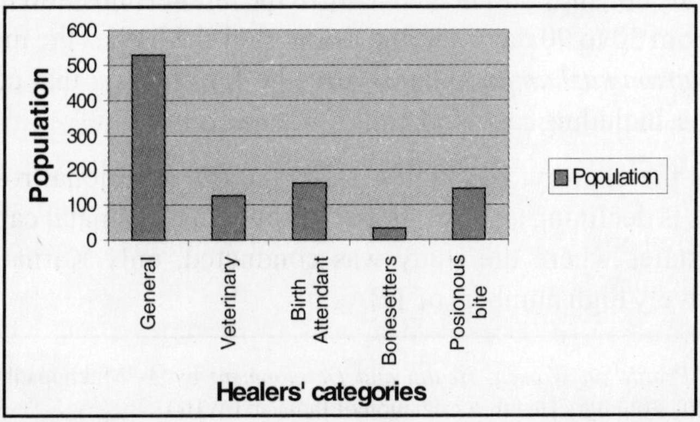

Traditional birth attendants

TBAs attend upon normal deliveries and form the largest group of specialised practitioners. Most rural deliveries are still taken care of by them. Their specialisation also includes prenatal and postnatal care, although they are usually called in near the time of delivery. Most TBAs belong to the lower social classes and communities in rural areas. The *Chakkiliyars, Ambattaiyars* and *Parayars* of Tamil Nadu and the *Kurubaru, Ambattaiya* and *Uppara* communities of Karnataka have a strong presence in this branch of traditional midwifery. In Kerala the midwives, known as *pettichi*, mainly belong to the barber and *Parayar* communities. Both come from a lower societal class. However, this trend seems to changing, with other communities also taking up this profession. It is possible that the training courses in midwifery that the government has recently initiated might have influenced this inflow from other communities.

Birth attendants are also a good source of information regarding medicinal preparations used in pre- and postnatal care. For example, *Nadamaruntu* is given to the mother in the days following delivery. This preparation, which contains many herbs and raw drugs collected from the *Nattumaruntu kadai* or raw drug shop, helps the mother regain her health more quickly. Medicinal preparations of this kind aim to improve the health of the nursing mother.

The care offered by these midwives does not stop at assisting in delivery; they also prescribe or provide neonatal care. It is not uncommon to see some of their practises become part of household traditions. In Kerala's tradition of postnatal care, the *pettichi* takes care of the mother and child for a period ranging from 30 to 90 days. During this period she bathes the mother with *Dhanvantaram kuzhampu* — an Ayurvedic formulation that contains 46 ingredients, including castor oil, milk, ghee and oil.

Across the country, especially in Kerala, the traditional role of birth attendants is declining and has shrunk to cover just postnatal care. Among the four states where the study was conducted, only Karnataka has a comparatively high numbers of TBAs.[47]

---

[47] *National Profile on Women, Health and Development* by A. Mukhopadhyay (2000). New Delhi: Voluntary Health Association of India and WHO.

Visa vaidyas — poisonous bite healers

During the survey, we found this group to be the second largest among the specialised traditional healers. These healers treat snakebites and poisonous stings, as well as administer antidotes for poisoning through ingestion.

As snakebites are life threatening, accurate diagnosis is crucial. The location of the bite, the colour of the wound, and physical and mental symptoms are all studied during the process of diagnosis. States of unconsciousness and hallucination are perceived to indicate a bad prognosis as they imply an advanced stage of poisoning. Other than bodily symptoms, other factors like signs and omens from nature and the environment are also taken into account during the healing process.

Poisons are generally classified into *vata, pitha* and *kapha.* For example, cobra venom is *vata*, but a viper's is *pitta.* In the *vata* type of poisoning, the patient exhibits a higher degree of neurological distress.

This branch of traditional healing is usually the first choice even in suburban areas, provided a healer is available. The transmission of this tradition follows particularly strict criteria. Courage and patience are two qualities that all healers stress when teaching apprentices. In most cases, the knowledge of healing connected to poisons is part of family traditions and is passed down from generation to generation. One reason for this could be that it demands an extraordinary degree of dedication.

The treatment for poisonous bites includes both internal and external medication, such as nasal drops, eye applications, and in some cases even purgatives. Many poisonous plants are also used, although after processing. The use of metals and minerals is also not rare.

Veterinary healers

The health of cattle and other livestock is given great importance by many communities whose livelihood depends on them. It is therefore not surprising that the maximum number of veterinary healers hail from cattle-rearing communities. For example, the *Kurubas* in Karnataka have a high number of veterinary practitioners. According to a report from one of our field locations (Chitradurga in Karnataka), the majority of healers in this area specialised in veterinary care.

These *vaidyas* manage a wide range of conditions, such as broken bones, communicable diseases (like foot and mouth), loose motions with blood, aversion to food, cough and so on. Most of these conditions are attributed to the ingestion of dirty grass, unhygienic conditions, infection from other cows, mud mixed with grass in the stomach, ingestion of polluted water, and chemicals in the grass and feed. Field experience shows that in the rural areas of Karnataka and Tamil Nadu, the first choice for veterinary care is the traditional veterinary healer. It is important to note in this context that of the 124 veterinary healers interviewed, most were over the age of 50 years.

Bonesetters

Bone setting is commonly practised in the rural and urban areas of southern India. Bamboo splints, white cotton cloth, egg and black gram powder are the main resources used in this branch of healing. Except for some families, the 34 bonesetters we met used natural medicinal resources very sparingly. And where medicinal oils and internal medications were used, it was not uncommon to find healers using their own formulae for them. Bone setting also appears to be male-dominated, though we did come across one exception: Muthukannu, a 45-year-old housewife from a farming family in Kovandakkurichi of Trichy District, who had learned this skill from her father in order to keep the family tradition alive.

The technique for bandaging differs from area to area. During the course of our study we came across a novel technique used by the bonesetters of Pudukkottai — that of using wooden channels to immobilise the leg. In many parts of southern India, traditional bonesetters use the verandas of shops for treating patients, but it is not rare to see them also operating in hospitals. Practitioners often refer patients to more experienced healers or hospitals in cases of severe trauma and open fractures.

General practitioners

A majority of healers fall under this category as they deal with both general ailments as well as specific, organ-related conditions. The category thus includes general practitioners, eye practitioners, spiritual healers, masseurs, *marma*[48] practitioners, etc.

[48] *Marma/varma* experts are *vaidyas* who specialise in treating traumatic problems and chronic problems of vital points in the body.

The practise of *Marma cikitsa*, a treatment based on the 107 vital points in the body, is found to be flourishing in Kerala and southern parts of Tamil Nadu. The treatment uses both internal and external medicines, with specialised massages and certain kinds of fracture reduction techniques also forming part of this tradition. To become a *marma* requires extensive training, and in Kerala this is usually given as part of the traditional martial art of *Kalari*.

Kannu vaidyam—the practice of eye medicine—that is a very specialised branch of traditional healing is not so prevalent though a few practitioners can still be found. In this tradition, both curative and promotive aspects of eye care are practised. *Anjanas* (collyriums) and eye drops are the main medications used in the treatment. The creation of a round-wall basin helps patients to retain the medicine (usually medicated oils and juices of herbs) in the eye. Surgical intervention in cataract is also practised by certain families, but is generally rare.

The younger generations in healing

Healing traditions are generally transmitted from generation to generation by word of mouth. Texts and palm leaf manuscripts are used to add to their knowledge during and after the training period under their *gurus*. This knowledge is passed on to select candidates based on the strict criteria mentioned earlier.

Unfortunately, the number of newcomers to the folk healing tradition is decreasing. According to one study, from among 1,000 *vaidyas*, about 671 were over 50 years old. Of these, only 38 per cent are continuing with healing as a family tradition.

Family traditions in healing

There are several families that have kept alive healing traditions that date back to several centuries. In the area of eye care, the Olagapuram Kannu *Vaidyar* family is well known. In some cases the tradition is unbroken and still alive in the hands of what are today the ninth and tenth generations. For instance, *Vaidya* Kathirvelar of Saaripudukkottai, Nallur, in Madurai District, claims to represent the thirty-first generation, while Kalvimadai Iyer, who treats poisonous bites and is practising *Jyotisi* (astrology), is twenty-first in the family tree of healers. A twelfth generation person from a birth attendant's family of Bettadanagenahalli, Bheemasamudra, (Chitradurga) still continues the service.

Support from manuscripts

Traditional healers update their knowledge by continually referring to the classical literature of Ayurveda and other regional manuscripts based on Ayurveda and Siddha. Documentation shows that 16 per cent of healers have a written source of knowledge in the form of textbooks or palm leaf manuscripts, many of which are rare.

Household Traditions of Health Management

Preventive, promotive, and curative health-related practises are visible in most homes and form an integral part of local lifestyles. Home remedies, health-related customs, food and regimens, all form part of the health tradition at the household level. For example, *moringa* leaves with pepper seeds or *jeera* along with *dal* is given to enhance breast milk; pepper *rasam* is often prescribed for cough and cold in southern India.

Health-related traditions at household level vary among ethnic communities and across regions. This was illustrated by the practises of the 2,000 households and 190 ethnic communities across 13 South Indian families analysed in our study. Often, these practises are associated with local belief systems. For example, during *Sankranti habba* (a harvest festival celebrated in Karnataka), there is a custom of distributing sesame seeds and jaggery to people. Apart from the belief that this is auspicious, it is believed to combat the common cold.

Home remedies are mostly curative and are the first intervention in domestic health problems. For instance, in southern India, *adhatodai* (*Adhatoda vasica*) leaves are used to treat cough and fever and *Sotru katralai* (*Aloe vera*) is used for cuts, wounds and uterine problems. Our study revealed that there are between 60 and 120 health conditions being managed at the domestic level. The local communities in Dakshina Kannada District, Karnataka, believe drinking a decoction made from the bark of *saptaparni*

(*Alstonia scholaris)* can prevent malaria. Some home remedies are very specific to ethnic communities. For instance, the Havyakka Brahmins consume *thambali* (a preparation made from ground coconut, curd and fried *sambar soppu* [*Coleus aromaticus*]) leaves for treating colds.

Region-specific recipes are also not uncommon. In Kerala, a porridge prepared from arrowroot powder and banana is given to babies as a nutrient. Sometimes, however, the same resources are used across regions for the same health problems. Many resources that go into treating gastric disturbances are used with a similar understanding in different regions. Cuts are treated with *arishina* or *manjal* or *haldi* powder (*Curcuma longa*), while *keelanelli* (*Phyllanthus amarus*) is used for curing jaundice. Some examples of health conditions managed at home are:

Table 6.2

Examples of Resources Used from the Kitchen for Home Remedies

Resource	Health condition	Area
1 Cumin	Cough, indigestion, burning micturition, fever	Kerala
2 Coriander	Indigestion, skin disease, throat pain,	Karnataka
3 Clove	Toothache	Kerala, Karnataka
4 Black pepper	Cold, cough	Karnataka, Kerala
5 Turmeric	Cuts and wounds	Karnataka, Kerala, Tamil Nadu
6 Ginger	Headache, indigestion	Karnataka, Kerala, Tamil Nadu

Many of the plants used come from kitchen gardens, farmlands or markets. Households generally prefer to use resources available in their vicinity and many home remedies use the same resources that are used in cooking. Spices and condiments are therefore widely utilised.

Most households use plant-based drugs rather than animal-based ones. Either the whole plant or parts of the plant finds use in remedies. For instance, leaves of *tulsi* are used to treat colds; seeds of fenugreek are used to treat diarrhoea, body ache; and the juice of a pomegranate is used as a coolant.

Home remedies are prepared using a single drug, or two to four. This makes it easier to prepare them in the household. The dosage forms include fresh juice, decoction and ground paste. As has been pointed out, more herbal medicines than those based on minerals and metals are prepared at home, probably because mineral and metal dosages require a high level of expertise.

Our study also showed that there is more than one remedy for a specific health condition and most households have an understanding of the efficacy of the drugs available. Alternatives and the availability of the resources in terms of seasonal variation is also a consideration. For example, vomiting can be controlled by either *omam* seeds (*Trachyspermum ammi*) or fresh lemons (*Citrus limon*). It could be inferred that due to seasonal variation, fresh lemons are not always available; a dry condiment like *omam*, on the other hand, can be stored and used off-season.

Aspects of food and regimen

Food and regimen play an important role in maintaining good health. Food and seasonal routines are considered as important as social well-being and spiritual factors in maintaining health. An understanding of food and activities that are unwholesome and wholesome (*apathya* and *pathya*) is therefore common. Avoiding the consumption of oily food during indigestion, brinjal in itching, or curds at night are some examples of *apathyas.* (i.e., practises to be avoided). Lighter food preparations, such as gruel in the case of fever, or eating pickles without oil and only a light seasoning along with food, are all *pathya* practises to be encouraged. The principle is also followed in seasonal food preparations and regimens. In the monsoon season (*karkata masa*), Keralites eat *karakada kanji* (a porridge prepared from red rice and medicinal herbs). This alleviates *vata* that tends to vitiate in this season.

Customs related to health

Health-related customs and beliefs are another aspect of health traditions at the household level. Religious practises, ceremonies, rituals and festivals related to seasonal changes are a few instances where customs and beliefs may be observed. For example, there are special customs related to puberty or pregnancy. Special nutritious foods like banana, *til* and jaggery sweets and food made with ghee are given during puberty. This is to provide the extra nutrition needed in this period of rapid growth. *Valakappu* or *baletodhisuvudu* is a common custom in southern India. Here, pregnant women are offered a green sari or dress, green bangles as well as flowers and fruits of their choice. This takes place in the seventh month during a ceremony in which the women in the family and other close friends participate. The custom is meant to reassure the woman of familial support and thereby give her mother confidence and courage.

Festivals related to seasons

Ramanavami is a festival celebrated during mid-summer in Karnataka. People usually fast on this day, consuming only those food items that are prepared with beaten rice and drinking *panakam* (prepared with the pulp of wood apple or musk melon combined with jaggery and tamarind). These items act as body coolants.

Conclusion

A range of LHTs was documented at household level in the study areas. Some examples of such traditions have already been provided. The action of revitalisation should start with a better understanding of the traditional practises in a systematic and comprehensive way. This makes a documentation exercise imperative. There are hundreds and thousands of practises that are part of the health care traditions of different communities. Many of these are still of contemporary relevance. The quantum of resources required for a comprehensive study on the health traditions of over 4000 communities will be huge. More micro-level initiatives will therefore be needed to tackle the issue of erosion, protection of intellectual property rights of the communities, and nurturing relevant practises to meet our growing primary health care needs.

Apart from documentation, another aim of our study was to ensure that practises considered effective by the communities continue to be promoted. The methodology used to do this is described in the next chapter.

7

A Participatory Approach in Assessing Health Traditions

A. Hafeel, T.S. Suma and P.M. Unnikrishnan

In Chapter 6 we described the first phase of the programme that the Foundation for Revitalisation of Local Health Traditions (FRLHT) initiated in 1998–2000. In this chapter, we focus on the second phase of the programme.

Phase –II: Rapid Assessment of LHTs (RALHT)

The objective in phase II was to develop a rapid assessment protocol to identify the best, most effective home remedies for the promotion of primary health care. In order to meet this objective, a series of five RALHT workshops were conducted in Kerala and Tamil Nadu. The exercise was called 'rapid' as it did not involve detailed laboratory or clinical studies and could be completed in a relatively short period of time.

We used a participatory approach to conduct this community-based assessment. The research group was multi-disciplinary and comprised local community members, folk healers, practitioners of Ayurveda, Siddha, Unani and Allopathy, as well as botanists and researchers. We based the assessment on the practical experience of local communities, supplementing it with the experiences of practitioners from the indigenous codified streams, who heal with the support of the classical literature of Ayurveda, Siddha and Unani, as well as other documented pharmacological findings.

Planning meeting on RALHT

As a prerequisite to RALHT protocol development, a workshop was conducted to finalise the methodology for assessing local health traditions (LHTs) at the household level. The participants were representatives of the Indian systems of medicine, public health and pharmacology. It was concluded that reference data would facilitate the respective experts in assessing practices. The formats for the assessment workshop and reference data collection on individual resources (plants, animals, minerals and metals) used were finalised for analysis by the respective systems of medicine. A format to record the communities' understanding of diseases, their management, cost feasibility and efficacy was also finalised. Subsequently, five areas were short-listed for assessment workshops from the 13 field collaborations. These areas were selected on the basis of completion of documentation and processing of data, as well as the diversity of practice and the quality of data.

Pre-workshop exercise

Prior to the RALHT workshop, a pre-workshop exercise was conducted, the main objective of which was to prioritise health conditions in the specific study areas selected for the assessment workshop. This was done through Participatory Rural Appraisal (PRA). Facilitated by trained field staff from several NGOs, the participants in this exercise consisted of about 20 to 35 respondents from the documentation phase.

The PRA exercise included the following five steps:

1 The listing of the health problems seen in their area by the community.
2 The prioritisation of important health problems from the list.
3 The listing of criteria used to prioritise the health conditions by the community.
4 The development of a matrix using the criteria and health conditions.
5 The ranking of health conditions (matrix ranking) based on each criterion.

Communities' understanding of the prioritised health conditions like causes, symptoms and stages were also discussed and documented. Health conditions that received the highest scores (ranging from 6 to 14) in each area were selected for assessment. These were then screened based on:

- availability of home remedies from the documented household data during Phase I
- remedies that were repeatedly mentioned during interviews
- accessibility of natural resources in the study area and the affordability of these resources

- remedies that are easy to prepare.

Based on the results, household remedies of specific areas were considered for assessment.

Literature references for the resources used

Natural resource (plant, animal, mineral) references for the selected plants were collected from the classical literature of Ayurveda, Siddha and Unani, as well as modern pharmacology, using the formats finalised during the protocol development meetings. This data served as the supportive documentation for commenting on the selected practises.

Selection of remedies

The following criteria were used to select the remedies for promotion:

1 Remedies for which there is strong and positive empirical evidence that is confirmed by the experience of local communities.

2 Consensus on efficacy by the multidisciplinary expert group or confirmation of efficacy by at least one ISM (Ayurveda, Siddha or Unani).

3 Remedies for which there is positive empirical evidence but are negatively assessed by all indigenous systems. These were selected for further community-based research and clinical studies.

The Workshop

Briefing sessions

On the day before the workshop, a session was held for rapporteurs[49] and facilitators to brief them on the methodology to be used for RALHT. On the same day, along with community members and local botanists, they were asked to collect voucher specimens of reported plant species for confirmation of their findings during the workshop.

On the day of the workshop, all participants were briefed on the Participatory Rapid Assessment of Local Health Traditions programme. Their role in the workshop was also outlined. This was done in separate sessions, one for

[49] The rapporteurs did the actual documenting.

the experts and one for the community. The formats for recording practices and comments were also explained to the expert groups.

Formation of working groups

Following the briefing sessions, different groups were formed, each with 12–20 members. Each group consisted of community members (households), a representative from Ayurveda, Siddha, Unani and Allopathy, two folk healers, a botanist, facilitator and two rapporteurs.

Discussions in the working groups

Each group facilitator presented the data documented on prioritised health conditions as well as the local remedies followed in households. The ensuing discussions covered mainly two aspects:

1 Communities' understanding of the health condition, its causes and symptoms.

2 Management of health conditions by households. This included details such as resources used and their confirmation using standard specimens, their proportion, preparation of medicines, dosage form, dosage and diet regulations, etc.

Using the structured format, rapporteurs documented the discussions of their respective working groups. After each working group completed discussing the parameters required, a plenary session was called wherein all the respective groups discussed the results or outcome of their exercise with others. Differences in opinion were clarified and a common understanding was reached.

Based on the five RALHT workshops, a methodology for rapid assessment evolved. About 50 remedies were assessed for 20 health conditions from three study areas in Tamil Nadu.

Analysis and Findings

The findings of a preliminary analysis of the complete process are presented below. This includes only the RALHT programmes in the three areas of Tamil Nadu (Trichy, Pondicherry, and Virudhunagar).

Table 7.1

Conditions Reported and Treated at Household Level

1	Abdominal pain during menstrual period	26	Different types of pain in the body
2	Anaemia/*Rathasokai*	27	Dhobi's itch
3	Back pain	28	Dry cough
4	Bleeding from the nose	29	Dryness in the skin
5	Bleeding gums	30	Dust falling in the eyes
6	Blood clots in minor trauma	31	Ear ache
7	Body itch	32	Ear discharge
8	Boils on the skin	33	Oedema of feet
9	Boils in the ear	34	Oedema of other body parts
10	Boils on the eyelids	35	Epilepsy
11	Breathing difficulty	36	Excess menstruation
12	Brittle teeth	37	Excess thirst
13	Burning eyes	38	Eyesight (to improve)
14	Burning micturition	39	Fever
15	Burning sensation in the legs	40	Fever, cough and cold
16	Chest pain	41	Foul smelling discharge
17	Chicken pox	42	Gas trouble
18	Cholera	43	General health promotion
19	Constipation	44	General weakness
20	Cough and cold in children	45	Giddiness
21	Cracks in the heel/feet	46	Greying hair
22	Cuts	47	Hair falling
23	Dandruff	48	Hair growth (to promote)
24	Delivery care	49	Headache
25	Diarrhoea in children	50	Heartburn

(contd.)

(Table 7.1 contd.)

51	Whooping cough	78	Piles
52	Indigestion	79	Productive cough
53	Indigestion/lack of appetite in cows	80	Redness in the eyes
54	Inflammation in the eyes	81	Running nose
55	Insect bite	82	Scorpion bite
56	Intestinal worms	83	Skin conditions in children
57	Irritation in the eyes	84	Skin rashes
58	*Janni* (type of fever)	85	Snakebite
59	Jaundice	86	Sneezing
60	Joint inflammation	87	Sores
61	Joint pain	88	Sour belching
62	*Kanvizhi*- (eye disorder)	89	Spider poisoning
63	Lack of appetite	90	Split hair
64	Lice	91	Sprain
65	Loose motions	92	Stomach pain
66	Loose motions with blood	93	Tastelessness
67	Loose motions with mucus	94	*Thalai pittham* – a type of headache
68	Malaria	95	Throat pain
69	Measles	96	To improve breast milk
70	Medicines in pregnancy	97	Toothache
71	Mouth ulcers	98	*Vata disorders*
72	Newborn care	99	*Vata neer* - *Vata* type of edema
73	Noise in the ear	100	Vomiting
74	One-sided headache	101	White discharge
75	Other diseases in the eyes	102	Wounds
76	Pain in micturition	103	Yellowish urine
77	Pain in the eyes		

Conditions reported from households

During our survey of the three areas, households reported 103 conditions that were partially or completely treated at the household level itself (see Table 7.1).

Natural resources used

The number of resources used in household health care range from 84 to 127. The maximum number of plant species was from the operational area

Table 7.2

Conditions and Formulae Assessed

Area code	No.	Condition	No. of remedies	Comments on remedies by different system of practice					
				LC	F	A	S	U	Allo
AURO	1	Common cold (Chali)	4	43	23 16 1 DD	43 O	4 DD	33 16	13 13 O 1 DD
	2	Dysentery	2	23	23	23 23 O	23	23	13 13 O
	3	Fever	3	33	23 1 DD	33	23 1 DD	23 13 O	13 13 O 1 DD
	4	Gas trouble	3	33	33	23 1 DD	33	23 13 O	3 DD
	5	Toothache	3	33	23 1 DD	23 13 O	33	23 13 O	3 DD
	6	White discharge	3	33	33	33	23 1 DD	33	3 DD
CCD	1	Head ache	3	33	33	3 DD	33	23 1 DD	3 DD

(contd.)

(Table 7.2 contd.)

Area code	No.	Condition	No. of remedies	Comments on remedies by different system of practice					
				LC	F	A	S	U	Allo
	2	Chest pain	1	13 O	13 O	1 DD	1 DD	13	13
	3	Dysmenorrhoea	2	13 13 O	13 13 O	2 DD	13 1 DD	13 1 DD	2 DD
	4	Janni	2	23	23	2 DD	2 DD	13 1 DD	16 1 DD
	5	Jaundice	1	13	13	13	13	13	13
	6	Eye pain	3	33	33	3 DD	26 1 DD	13 1 DD 16	26 1 DD
	7	Burning sensation of the eye	3	33	33	3 DD	33	13 23 O	231 DD
	8	Menorrhagia	2	133 O	23	13 1 DD	13 13 O	23	13 1 DD
	9	Tooth ache	4	43	33 1 DD	4 DD	23 2 DD	23 2 DD	4 DD
	10	Gas trouble	3	33	33	3 DD	33	33	23 1 DD
	11	Scabies/skin condition	3	33	23 1 DD	13 O 2 DD	33	33	13 2 DD
ANSA	1	Common cold	2	23	23	23	23	13 1 DD	2 DD
	2	Indigestion in children	2	23	23	2 DD	23	2 DD	23
	3	General itching	3	23 13 O	23 13 O	13 2 DD	13 13 O 1 DD	23 1 DD	3 DD

(contd.)

(Table 7.2 contd.)

Area code	No.	Condition	No. of remedies	Comments on remedies by different system of practice					
				LC	F	A	S	U	Allo
	4	Jaundice	2	23	23	23	1 3 13 O	13 O 1 DD	13 13 O
	5	Migraine	2	23	23	23 O	13 1 DD	2 DD	13 1 DD
	6	Piles	2	23	23	23 O	13 1 DD	13 1 DD	2 DD
	7	Stomachache	3	23 13 O	13 23 O	13 23 O	13 23 O	13 23 O	1 DD 23 O
	8	Vomiting	3	33	23 13 O	23 13 O	33	13 2 DD	3 DD
	9	White discharge	2	23	23	23	23	13 1 DD	2 DD

Notes:

3 - Effective remedy

O - Should be used with modification specified by the group

6 - Should not be advocated and are not effective

DD - Data deficient/unable to comment

of an NGO, i.e., the Covenant Centre for Development. The materials used in home remedies also include 32 resources of animal origin and 19 of mineral origin. Forty-four per cent of plant species used in home remedies were available locally.

Learnings from the Exercise

The presence of a strong, local group of experts (healers who are experts in terms of their experience in health care and their familiarity with the vernacular language) is vital. This would enable a fruitful interaction between community members and representatives of other systems of medicine. A committed and sensitive expert group is also essential to ensure the best results for the entire exercise; they should therefore be carefully selected. The consensus is that their selection should be based on the following criteria:

1 Openness towards LHTs and revitalisation initiatives.

2 Proficiency in the vernacular language.

3 Being local, with experience in working in the same area/community.

4 Willingness to spend time with the local community for the workshop.

5 Technical proficiency (ability to translate or explain the conditions or practises as per his/her knowledge stream after enough interaction with the community).

6 Folk healers should be locally accepted healers.

7 A folk healer with more than 10 years experience in the health care of the local area would be ideal.

In the pre-workshop exercise, we found it was more profitable to discuss priority areas in the presence of local folk healers. This helps in achieving a better understanding of the community's health conditions from the health worker's point of view. It also enables a better survey of the available literature on these health conditions. Therefore, an orientation seminar for local healers is a must. This must be organised prior to the workshop in order to ensure the objectivity of their contribution. Similarly, briefing participants from other systems of medicine is important as a sensitising exercise.

During the pre-workshop exercise, data regarding health conditions should be collected in detail. It is also essential to limit the number of health conditions and formulae to be assessed per day in order to facilitate a complete and comprehensive discussion. With regard to the preparation of reports and developing an action-oriented package, we learned that a decentralised method for processing workshop outputs would yield more accurate data. Confirmation and standard specimen referrals (with a proper correlation of local and binomial names) for backing up data should also be completed as part of the workshop sessions. Fine-tuning the documentation phase in terms of sampling, modification of questionnaires and additional inputs in capacity building for field staff are also essential.

In many instances, ISM physicians make comments on a recipe based on the property of individual drugs. It may not be always possible to judge the efficacy of such a formulation, as there could be changes when ingredients are combined. The efficacy of a combination in such situations can be understood only through a detailed clinical study.

Confining the PRA process to curative practises can lead us to overlook many important preventive and promotive practises, which are equally relevant aspects of LHTs. An example is practise of drinking *Mukkudi kashaya* to enhance production of breast milk; in Kerala, *Karkidaka kanji* is imbibed during the rainy season to prevent rheumatic complaints. It is thus essential to have preset criteria or thematic discussions on these aspects during such exercises.

According to the expert groups who reviewed the process, some of the practises assessed through the rapid method should also undergo a process of rapid clinical trials in the rural set-up, with the active involvement of folk healers, communities and ISM practitioners. This process should record the individual experience of the community. It was also suggested that assessed remedies, which lacked sufficient data regarding properties or action or support from the ISM stream, be given priority during clinical trials.

In addition, it was felt that the RALHT process needed to be more local and decentralised if locality-specific problems and practises were to be given priority. We had restricted ourselves to the NGO set-up. It is necessary, therefore, to develop a locality-specific promotional strategy and build it into the RALHT process.

RALHT workshops have helped the community gain exposure to different areas of knowledge related to causes and symptoms. This has led to a better understanding of health, especially in the areas of prevention. The current understanding of the causes as well as symptoms of each condition at the household level is insufficient. For instance, a community from Virudhunagar believed that leprosy was caused by snakebite. This exercise gave the local community an opportunity to learn more about the causes, symptoms, and transmission of leprosy with the help of folk healers and ISM and Western medicine practitioners.

Mainstreaming the Findings

The Kitchen Herbal Garden (KHG) is one of the programmes that the FRLHT has initiated to promote positively assessed practises. In this programme, the PRA–RALHT process is used to promote a comprehensive package of medicinal plants for selected conditions at the household level. The RALHT process is mandatory to identify the conditions that need to be addressed through the KHG package. The attempt is to prioritise locally available solutions. It is now felt that a thematic PRA process could not only elaborate the scope of the programme by including the preventive and promotive aspects of LHTs, but also enhance local health customs and traditions. Fifteen field collaboration agencies have promoted positively assessed traditions using the RALHT methodology via home gardens. In 2001, 16,000 Kitchen Herbal Gardens were established in Tamil Nadu, Karnataka and Kerala (see Chapter 8 for further details of the KHG programme).

Recently, the RALHT methodology and our findings were presented at a forum of scientists and policymakers representing the central and state governments. Development NGOs were also present at this meeting held in Chennai on 22 January 2001. The objective was to formulate a strategy to promote positively assessed traditions, as well as the RALHT methodology, through both government and non-government programmes.

There exists a network of 13 NGOs that are already involved in the ex situ conservation of medicinal plants. Each of these NGOs has a medicinal plant conservation park that consists of a herbarium, a seed bank, a raw drug museum, an ethno-medicinal forest, and a nursery of medicinal plants used by healers and households in that area. Different interactive activities are organised by these NGOs with the help of local communities, local healers, ISM practitioners, botanists and others interested in the conservation of medicinal plants. Some of these centres even have clinics involving local healers and ISM practitioners.

Information gathered in the process of documentation is being utilised for improving the local resource centre in each of these areas. Currently, these centres operate as informal, LHT information centres; it is hoped that they will also serve as biodiversity repositories for the people.

In order to encourage other NGOs to take up the documentation and revitalisation of local health traditions, the RALHT methodology is being developed into a training module that could be used by both GOs and NGOs. Apart from an introduction to LHTs, the module provides training on documentation and identification of best practises by using a participatory rapid approach. Computer software has also been developed to digitalise data on LHTs. This helps NGOs organise and present documented data, which can be used as the health component of the people's biodiversity register.

We are currently engaged in conducting rapid clinical studies on some of the practises assessed during the RALHT. The intention is to generate further substantiating data to back our findings.

People's Knowledge and Ethics

One outcome of the documentation and assessment process has been the development of regional databases by the 13 centres. A local committee to support the revitalisation process has been also formed in each of these centres. It consists of folk healers, panchayat (local governing body) members, teachers of the locality and community leaders, and will be responsible for further utilisation of the data. Since the database is the intellectual property of the local community, it will be returned to the respective communities once the correction exercise is completed.

The formats for documenting each of the categories, as well as the database, will be used to promote the documentation of LHTs through panchayats, NGOs and other agencies. This will be done through a series of training programmes and will form the health component of the People's Biodiversity Registers, which contain extensive documentation of the local natural resources and their utilisation. Such registers are now being promoted in many parts of India. One objective of this programme is to protect local knowledge from being pirated for commercial purposes without the proper consent of local communities, or without any agreement for the equitable sharing of profits with the communities.

Conclusion

Exploring existing health practises, identifying and nurturing the best among them, adding to the incomplete aspects of these practises and discouraging their distortion — these are the four inevitable facets of any revitalisation process. The process envisaged by the RALHT encourages all four.

A more refined methodology that incorporates learnings from the RALHT workshops would have a great deal to offer NGOs involved in identifying and strengthening these traditions. As household traditions are very vast and diverse, repeating the process in each area would be a herculean task. It would thus be ideal if the RALHT process were to be replicated in a more localised and decentralised manner. In this context, the replication would have to be carried out with the involvement of different sectors of health care and cover various aspects of the health traditions, such as food habits, seasonal regimens, mother and child health care, and the specialised practises of healers.

It is also necessary to formulate locally compatible strategies for the wider promotion of best practises. Encouraging the cultivation of kitchen herbal gardens is one such strategy. In addition, the use of publications and effective communication through the media and NGOs should be pursued.

Currently, there is complete political apathy coupled with a discouraging social attitude towards this field, which is abundantly reflected in present-day health education/research/promotion programmes. These founts of local knowledge and local resource dependent practices have a definite and crucial role to play in achieving health for all. A pluralistic promotional strategy, which recognises and incorporates local expertise, is urgently needed. Chapter 8 shows how this can be done in one particular area, that of kitchen herbal gardens.

8

Health at Our Doorstep[50]
Reviving Home Remedies

G. Raju and G. Hariramamurthy

Millions of rural households use a large number of herbal home remedies and diets as part of their health care. The contribution of local health traditions (LHTs) to health care is a significant one. Knowledge and use of these by ethnic communities across the 600,000 villages of India today is critically dependent on access to and availability of plant resources across different eco-systems. This continuity needs to be preserved, as about 4,600 Indian ethnic communities know of and depend on about 8,000 out of a total of 15,000 flowering plants for their health care needs.[51] It is therefore an issue that warrants serious national and international attention. Easy access to plants is no longer as common as it used to be and under these circumstances, it is not surprising that local health traditions are being rapidly eroded. Unfortunately, there are hardly any government or non-government institutions working to keep this tradition alive.

Equally important is another issue: during eight five-year plan periods, both the central and state governments in India were able to provide only 3–4 per cent of their annual financial resources to meet the health care needs

---

[50] The authors deeply acknowledge the contribution made in the implementation of the Operation Health at the Door Step Programme to the following: the NGOs. Anthodaya Sangha (ANSA), Covenant Centre for Development (CCD), Gandeepam, Social Change and Development (SCAD), People's Agricultural Farm (PAF), League for Education and Development (LEAD), the Peoples' Federations, the Village Resource Persons, *nattu* vaidyars, Siddha doctors, schoolteachers, Kitchen Herbal Garden growers, Anantanarayana Sarma: rural management expert, Lakshmi Rehmatullah and her associates from Arvind Eye Hospital, Madurai, and other colleagues from FRLHT.

[51] 'A Green Pharmacy' by D. Shankar, D. K. Ved and U. G. Geetha (2000). *Hindu Folio*, October, pp. 14–17.

of the people.[52] Of this, only 0.5 to 3 per cent was allocated to Indian systems of medicine. The government public health services use their resources mostly to meet the salary-related costs of Allopathic doctors and paramedical staff.

According to Dr C. R. Chandrashekar (of the National Institute of Mental Health and Neuro-Sciences in Bangalore),[53] the State Government of Karnataka is able to allocate only an annual budget of Rs 30,000 per Primary Health Centre (PHC) for the purchase of medicines. With population coverage of 30,000 per PHC, this means that only medicines worth Re 1 per person per year is available to our citizens. Dr Prakash Rao of Drug Action Forum has pointed out that the public health services do not cover 80 per cent of the rural population, and that a large part of both public and private health services are urban-centred.

The Foundation for Revitalisation of Local Health Traditions (FRLHT), along with other non-governmental organisations, has been promoting the use of local health traditions, through a Medicinal Plants Conservation Programme. Under this programme, NGOs develop educational medicinal plant gardens complemented by a herbarium, and a raw drug and seeds museum. There is also an outreach component that focuses mainly on rural households to promote the growing and use of medicinal plants for both health and income-generation purposes. This activity has taken the shape of kitchen herbal gardens (KHGs) to be nurtured by rural households. The KHG package is meant to serve as a first response to a simple health problem that may occur in the household. Begun in 1997 as an integral part of the medicinal plants conservation programme, KHG was expected to demonstrate the contemporary relevance of self-reliance in primary health care.

Many NGOs are now implementing this programme through self-help groups (henceforth referred to as *sanghas*) of 20 women each. The NGOs

---

52 'Indigenous Health Services: The State of the Art' by D. Shankar (1992) in Alok Mukhopadhyay (ed.) *State of India's Health.* New Delhi: Voluntary Health Association of India.

53 Remarked during his presidential remarks in the afternoon session of the Karnataka Janarogya Sabhe (Karnataka State-level People's Health Assembly) in Davangere on 26 November 2000.

train the women in the use of medicinal plants for health applications and also provide a set of saplings that can be grown in and around the home. FRLHT has also developed a manual on medicinal plants in primary health care and some 20 plants have been chosen based on the experience of traditional *vaidyas*.

Initially, irrespective of where the NGOs were located, the same set of plants was being promoted in the KHGs. But a review of KHG activity, undertaken in early 1999, revealed that:

1 The uniform package was inappropriate due to differences in the availability of medicinal plants in the villages. Also, the health conditions prioritised by rural households were different in different locations.

2 The activity focused more on plants than on health conditions. Thus, in practise, NGOs were raising plants of their choice and convenience rather than plants that were appropriate for local health conditions.

3 Lack of planning and clarity of purpose rendered the unit cost of KHGs (which amounted to over Rs 1,000) unviable at the household level.

4 The scale of outreach was too small and not commensurate with the number of staff available at NGOs.

Based on the review, it was decided that:

- Promotional activity for KHG needed to be increased.
- This activity must result in KHGs being set up at rural households.
- Training and communication must focus on this outcome.
- The promotion of KHGs need not be restricted only to *sangha* members. The *sanghas* themselves could become vehicles for promoting KHGs in the villages they operate.
- The choice of medicinal plants would be based on health conditions prioritised by the local communities and take into account species that are available.

It was decided to use the participatory rural appraisal (PRA) methodology to determine the health conditions prioritised by local rural households. To this end, trainings were organised to help NGO staff develop skills in using this method. In the course of these training programmes it was discovered that:

- Rural households were already using some medicinal plants for domestic health conditions;
- Most communities had elders who were quite knowledgeable about the use of medicinal plants;
- The availability of medicinal plants within the village premises had some influence on the final choice of plants;
- Rural households were willing to pay for the plants, provided they were of their choosing.

In Thiruvallur colony in Thirunelveli district, Tamil Nadu, the PRA transect walk revealed that medicinal plants could be accessed from roadsides, storage ponds, farms, grasslands and wastelands. The people in the colony identified some plants (*kilanelli, kuppaimeni, sirianangai*, *avarampoo*, *arukampul*, *pirandai,* etc.) that were available in these habitats, as well as the seasons during which they could be accessed. This meant that the KHGs in that area would have to provide for plants other than these.

The experience of the PRA exercises confirmed that the KHG focus would have to shift from plants to health conditions, given that the people were easily able to identify health conditions and relate them to the necessary plants. It was therefore decided that the project would first identify health priorities and then select the medicinal plants to be grown in the KHGs, saplings for which would be provided for a fee. It was also decided that training would focus on the use of these plants for local health conditions. In this context, training strategies would need to take into account the availability of knowledgeable people in the village, who commanded the respect of the community, and establish linkages with them. In practise, this meant that resource persons for training would not need to be confined only to NGO staff.

The KHG programme was scaled up in the following year. Local resource persons were now used to provide training inputs on self-help home remedies.

A quantitative study, undertaken to assess the impact of the KHG programme on households that had participated in the programme in 1999–2000, revealed that people found the programme to be useful. Further, nearly three-fourths of the households that had set up KHGs knew the names of at least five medicinal plants and their uses, and had used at least one to two plants to treat health care problems.

The majority of the households interviewed were willing to pay, or were paying, for the seedlings of medicinal plants that were being supplied by nurseries managed by the medicinal plants conservation parks (MPCPs).

More importantly, the process of people-to-people extension was evident: on their own initiative, a number of households had started adding local medicinal plants to their gardens. They had also begun to share their knowledge and plant materials with neighbouring households.

When the findings of the study were shared in the review meeting, the NGOs and FRLHT decided that further up-scaling would be required to bring down the cost. Based on the findings, the KHG target for 2000–01 was raised to the establishment of 50,000 kitchen gardens.

Operation 'Health at Your Doorstep'

From 2000–2001, the KHG project acquired a new name: 'Operation Health at Your Doorstep'. Five NGOs in southern Tamil Nadu expressed willingness to execute the operation. It involved increasing the previous year's target by a factor of three. The rural management consultant, who had conducted the study in 1999–2000, was asked to provide extensive inputs to the NGOs, while FRLHT appointed a task force leader to coordinate the entire operation. The operation required that:

- The NGOs lay stress on the 'people-to-people process' by which growers and other local resource persons become extension agents for promoting KHGs to new growers. The NGOs' role then becomes one of planning, coordination and facilitation.
- The unit cost per KHG is brought down to Rs 70 (Rs 40 for training and Rs 30 for the supply of the 20 plant saplings).

- KHG growers pay for the cost of saplings.
- Focus is on the health conditions prioritised by KHG growers; this would help determine the choice of saplings to be grown.
- Training of village resource persons (VRPs) forms a key part of the process.

The process and methodology followed in the operation is the same for all NGOs.[54] The highlights of the process include regular monthly meetings around a key issue, documentation and follow-up action, regular visits by the management consultant to the NGOs for follow-up on outcomes of meetings, and stocktaking at the NGO level. Monthly meetings cover such issues as setting up of KHG targets, selection of species, planning and implementation of nurseries, training strategy, course development, identification of VRPs, and the costing for nurseries, training, database development, baseline surveys.

The following case study of the NGO *Gandeepam* outlines the strategy it used for its training programme and its outcome.

Gandeepam

Gandeepam was established as a registered society in 1991 under the Tamil Nadu Societies Act of 1975 in Sivagangai district of Tamil Nadu. Its six-point programme includes the conservation of medicinal plants and their sustainable utilisation, the promotion of community health based on the Siddha system of medicine, sustainable agriculture, empowerment of women, child rights and welfare, as well as poverty alleviation. However, it is in the first two areas that *Gandeepam* has carved out a name for itself. *Gandeepam*'s Medicinal Plants Conservation Park (MPCP) is situated in Kilavayal village in S. Pudur revenue block of Sivagangai district. Due to its location, it works in the revenue blocks of S. Pudur and Singampunari in Sivagangai district, as well as in the bordering revenue blocks of other districts like Marungapuri in Tiruchi, Natham in Dindigul, Kottampatti in Madurai and Ponnamaravathi in Pudukkottai. *Gandeepam* is one of the partners implementing the programme of medicinal plant conservation and sustainable utilisation coordinated by the

[54] The five NGOs are ANSA (Tiruchi), Gandeepam (Sivagangai), PAF (Pudukottai), SCAD (Tirunelveli) and CCD (Virudhunagar) in Tamil Nadu.

FRLHT. The KHG programme is targeted at 12,000 households in seven blocks distributed over five districts.

Each cluster of villages that participates in the KHG program has a core coordination group, which is responsible for the programme. Each of these groups has the benefit of a *naatu vaidyar* (a knowledgeable woman) assisting women leaders in the process. The groups have formulated a package of plants that are required for preparing home remedies. Based on the output of PRA exercises, 20 unique medicinal plants, including a few plants of nutritional importance, have been listed. The groups used this list to plan for nurseries; based on this, it was decided to raise and supply 240,000 seedlings within six months, keeping in mind the need to begin supplying seedlings to KHG households just prior to the onset of the monsoon, i.e., before September 2000, in order to ensure a higher survival rate for the plants. Later, the groups again met to draw up a time-activity chart, which essentially meant planning various activities across the 12 Tamil calendar months, as well as fixing a monthly physical target. This action plan was to cover an outreach target of 12,000 KHG households in 334 villages and hamlets distributed across five districts.

After launching the programme, the members of the core resource team met once a week at the block level and once a month at the central level to monitor and review progress. They also distributed among themselves the responsibility of achieving the annual targets. This was done based on the block-level assessments given by the members of respective block-level committees in consultation with the leaders of the women's *sanghas* of the various blocks. The KHGs developed in each location numbered: S. Pudur 2,500, Singampunari 2,500, Tirupathur 500, Marungapuri 6,000, Natham 500, Kottampatti 250, and Ponnamaravathi 250.

The core resource team also distributed the responsibility for specific tasks among its members with respect to various activities:

- scheduling and coordinating village-level Siddha health camps and demonstrations of KHGs
- identification and training of Village Resource Persons (VRPs)

Table 8.1

List of Medicinal Plants Given as Part of KHG Package

S no.	Botanical names of plants used as single or main ingredients	Diseases/ailments/conditions treated
1	*Adhatoda vasica*	Cough, white discharge, fever with cold
2	*Hibiscus rosa-sinensis*	Fever due to exhaustion, irregular or excess menstruation
3	*Lawsonia inermis*	Boils, cracked heels
4	*Centella asiatica*	Fever with cold and cough, memory increaser
5	*Murraya koenigii*	Gastric trouble, early greying
6	*Aloe vera*	Piles, eyesores, conjunctivitis, cuts and wounds
7	*Solanum trilobatum*	Cold, cough
8	*Punica granatum*	Dysentery, diarrhoea
9	*Andrographis alata*, *Andrographis ovata*	Swelling due to poisonous bites, itching
10	*Eclipta alba*	Dhobi itch, fungal skin infection, liver toner, hair growth
11	*Citrus limon*	Excess body heat, excess pitha, earache
12	*Coleus aromaticus*	Cough, fever with cold
13	*Solanum surattense*	Toothache
14	*Psidium guajava*	Dysentery
15	*Phyllanthus emblica*	Mouth ulcer, excess *pitha*
16	*Azadirachta indica*	Boils, fever, deworming
17	*Andrographis paniculata*	Poisonous bites – as first aid
18	*Alpinia galanga*	Cold, cough
19	*Tylophora asthmatica*	Asthmatic cough
20	*Enicostemma littorale*	White discharge

- establishment of demo-gardens and sharing of successful cures by the VRPs
- collection of advance payments from the KHG households
- collection of balance amounts from the KHG households
- village-level training-cum-demonstration of home remedy preparations for prioritised conditions
- preparations for establishing KHGs in households
- delivery of medicinal plants from the nursery
- establishment of KHG
- refresher training courses on self-help method.
- monitoring the performance of VRPs and the usage of KHG package by households, and providing solutions to problems that might arise.

As mentioned earlier, the core resource team, in consultation with women *sangha* leaders, had already determined the mode of operation to be adopted by the campaign, which was initiated in April 2000. It divided itself into five groups of five members each to conduct village-level Siddha camp-cum-demonstration of KHGs in the villages identified by them. Every evening at 4.00 p.m., four teams (each including one *nattu vaidyar* and one block-level staff member) leave the MPCP on their two-wheelers along with the requisite logistics for the health camp and demonstration. All four travel in four different directions. Two VRPs, respectively representing the block and village concerned, join the team en route or meet them in the village itself. Prior to their arrival, a volunteer would already have reached the village to ensure that all preparations for the demonstration-cum-camp were in order.

Each camp begins with a cultural event comprising songs and skits built around the theme of local health traditions and at every demonstration a live KHG plant package is kept on display for the participants. The demonstration of medicinal preparations and use of home remedies is done by the respective VRP from the particular village. The *nattu vaidyar* helps in clarifying any doubts raised by villagers; he also provides treatment for conditions that are difficult to treat with home remedies. The *nattu vaidyar* also explains and demonstrates how to prepare the medicine and administer it. If necessary, medicines produced by the *vaidyar* in the medicinal production unit located in the Gandeepam campus are sold to the patients. By the end of the day, the sale of medicines by the *nattu vaidyars* and their assistants fetch an income of Rs 1,000 to Rs 2,000.

After the demonstration, the live plants are used by the VRP of the village to actually establish a demo-garden, either in her own or neighbour's household. Thus, the village demo-cum-camps have already resulted in the establishment of four demonstration KHGs, a list of names of women interested in the KHG package, and a token advance amount of at least Rs 5 for the KHG plants to be supplied later.

Gandeepam also initiated a residential training programme for 750 VRPs identified by them. Following monthly review meetings between the coordinators and NGO staff in the Medicinal Plants Conservation Park of People's Agricultural Farm, and an NGO in the neighbouring district of Pudukkottai to discuss various aspects of the training, the core resource team of Gandeepam decided to provide a 20-hour residential training for its VRPs.

These trainings are conducted over two days, and cover different aspects of know-how and 'do-how' of KHG in six sessions. The training inputs include both classroom as well as practical working sessions. Training begins with a visit to the disease-based thematic garden in the MPCP campus, and each VRP is given a printed manual on how to prepare self-help home remedies.

The training also focuses on the establishment and maintenance of the KHG. During the training, VRPs are often asked to discuss common problems, such as cattle grazing and water scarcity, that can affect the survival of plants in KHGs, as well as demonstrate the use of practical measures to address such problems. Participants are required to establish a model KHG, with proper fencing and the use of different types of local materials, either within the MPCP campus or in a nearby village. (In areas where there is water scarcity, they also demonstrated how to use water from the kitchen/bathroom for nurturing the plants.) This also involves all the procedures to be followed before and after planting, i.e., digging pits of the correct size and filling it with the correct mixture of manure, soil and sand, mulching, watering and weeding.

Participants are simultaneously provided the opportunity to practically demonstrate the preparation of home remedies. Each of the five to six prioritised diseases is given a time slot of 30–60 minutes. At the end of each slot, the VRPs are asked to identify and collect the necessary plants or raw drug parts from the model KHGs and then demonstrate the preparation of medicinal formulations, i.e., hot/cold extraction, decoction, oils, pastes and powders.

Another important aspect of the campaign is its focus on gender. At least two to three topics covered by the training are health concerns prioritised by women, with sessions relating to these being conducted by women trainers (who discuss their doubts with the elderly *nattu vaidyars*, when and if necessary).

The involvement of competent and experienced *nattu vaidyars* and Siddha physicians as resource persons for the training is an important strategy. The pre-assessment and post-training evaluation exercises, conducted before and after the training programmes, help to determine the VRPs' needs, plan the level of inputs the training would provide, and confirm the transfer and assimilation of knowledge and skills during and at the end of each training session.

The block-level team also facilitates parallel exposure visits for village women from a new village to a neighbouring village where the KHG programme has been initiated in the previous year. The coordinator of the KHG programme, along with the concerned VRPs and staff members, accompany the villagers during such visits to facilitate people-to-people interaction and provide on-the-spot clarifications of any doubts raised by the visiting women.

The role of VRPs is critical for the success of the campaign. It is through these local women that the KHG package of training and plants is being delivered to other village women. The VRPs were drawn mainly from the leaders of women self-help groups engaged in micro-credit. After completing our training, the VRPs listed their role and responsibilities, along with a time-activity chart, for the following areas:

- the establishment of a demonstration model of KHG in their own household premises;
- the sharing of successful cures of medicinal plants from their model KHG to demonstrate its use to other households in the village;
- village-level training-cum-preparations for prioritised conditions;
- preparations for establishing KHGs in households, i.e., fencing, laying of a wastewater channel, pitting, and the mixing of sand, soil and manure;
- collection of advance payments from KHG households;
- delivery of medicinal plants;
- establishment of KHGs by households;
- refresher training on self-help home remedies;
- collection of balance amounts from KHG households;
- monitoring of the usage of the KHG package.

Thirty-six-year old Ms Chandra is one of the 750 VRPs enlisted in the programme. She is a block-level resource person from her village (Pullampatti in Sivagangai district) and is also one of the 36 core committee members. Her family comprises of herself, her husband and three children. They have a small landholding of around half-an-acre. The couple manages to earn an average monthly income of Rs 900 for 10 months in a year, mostly by making coir ropes from coconut fibre and weaving thatches from coconut leaves. During the two peak months of summer, they manage to survive by collecting and selling *neem* seeds. Her village is located at the tail end of the district bordering Trichy, which was once known for the brewing of country liquor. With the initiation of awareness activities under the adult literacy and KHG programmes, this has now been halted. Three years ago, she initiated the first women micro-credit *sangha* in her village; her perseverance and diligence led to the formation of a second one, and now a third *sangha* is about to be formed. Her most valuable contribution lies in extending the KHG concept to the neighbouring villages of Musinthapatti, Thimmalaikudi, Vijayapuram, Mettampatti, Kulathupatti, Perumalpatti and Vadakadu, which she did through person-to-person interaction. She and a few other *sangha* leaders invited the women of other villages to visit theirs, and see the KHGs established by her and her neighbours. After the visit and the discussions that took place between the women, the KHG programme was also extended to the other villages.

While speaking of the contribution that the KHG programme has made to their lives, Ms Chandra said:

> "While promoting the revitalisation and use of our knowledge and plants to address our health needs, the Kitchen Herbal Garden programme has also taught us that money not spent is money saved. We now spend less on our family's medical treatment and hence are able to save more than earlier. I spent Rs 55 for getting the plants for my KHG garden. But, I also managed to earn Rs 60 in the year by supplying plant materials to the nursery."

The KHG package of plants promoted by her and other VRPs in her block contains 20 plants comprising 14 species. On her own initiative, she has added the *Hibiscus rosa sinensis, Aloe vera, Ocimum sanctum*, *Nochi* and *Nethrapoondu* to the package. She has also supplied cuttings of hibiscus, *Adhatoda vasica*, *Eclipta alba* and *Lawsonia inermis* to the nursery of a neighbouring MPCP of the Covenant Centre for Development. MsChandra regularly uses plants from the KHG for her own family's health needs, as well as for her neighbours.

Linking KHG with Household Economic Activity

Sanjivini (which means 'eternal life') is a federation of women's self-help groups with 7,000 women members and is engaged in micro-credit and micro-enterprise activities. Sanjivini has introduced a novel scheme under the KHG programme. Under this scheme, KHG households are not only trained to grow and use medicinal plants for the needs of their own families, but are also encouraged to supply a few medicinal plants, such as *Adhatoda vasica* and *Eclipta alba*, to the medicine manufacturing unit, which is managed and run by local folk health practitioners. (The monthly turnover of the unit is around Rs 30,000.) SHGs involved in the KHG programme had collected *neem* seeds during the last summer and processed them to obtain the medicinal *neem* oil (used in their homes for de-worming), as well as *neem* oil and cake for agricultural and other purposes. Thus, for these women, conserving the diversity of medicinal plants also has value in economic terms.

As a follow-up to the programme, the FRLHT has also initiated an impact survey on the KHG programme in eight districts of Tamil Nadu (Tuticorin, Tirunelveli, Virudhunagar, Sivagangai, Pudukottai, Trichy, Perambalur, Karur). Here, the KHG programme is being implemented by five MPCPs using a people-to-people extension strategy.

The survey is meant to help the implementing NGOs to:

1 assess the impact of the KHG programme and its usage by the households covered
2 find and understand village-level variables that positively or negatively influence the implementation of the KHG programme in the villages covered
3 find and understand the household-level variables that positively or negatively influence decision-making with respect to the use of home remedies as the first response to simple ailments.

Though the KHG project was originally initiated as an integral part of the medicinal plants conservation programme, it was decided to continue the package as an ongoing, independent programme. It was also accepted that for KHG to succeed as a strategy for promoting local health traditions, the project would have to offer KHG adopters some tangible benefits, such as the enabling the resource-poor rural households to save on health expenses. It was also felt that since the programme had become self-driven and self-sustaining, with NGOs facilitating the process of decentralising the implementation of the KHG package through village-level resource persons, its actual implementation should be given over to people's institutions. The NGOs and women's self-help groups and their federations were therefore given necessary training inputs for capacity building to achieve a critical mass by upscaling the KHG programme.

The first round of the benchmark survey[55] that was completed in May

[55] Report on KHG Bench Mark Study by A. Sharma and Lakshmi Rahmathulla (2001). Bangalore: Foundation for Revitalisation of Local Health Traditions. Unpublished.

2001 has been able to confirm that the KHG package:

- was adopted by non-*sangha* members (44 percent) with equal interest, though it was implemented through women's self-help groups (56 percent)
- was adopted more easily by small, nuclear families (64 percent) with 5–6 members; large joint families were less enthusiastic
- was readily received by a majority of the households (76 percent) belonging to poor or very poor rural families
- was biased in favour of the traditionally disadvantaged and socially and economically backward sections (100 percent) of society
- was willingly adopted by women (100 percent)
- was accepted (100 percent) as a first response to a primary health care problem at the household level
- was fully paid for by 90 percent of KHG households
- was known to a large number of the rural communities and used in local health traditions. Nearly 35 percent of KHG households planted medicinal plants on their own initiative. About 68 percent of KHG households confirmed that they knew of plant-based home remedies before adopting the package
- was believed by nearly 93 percent as offering effective cures for simple health problems
- could be extended beyond the actual KHG households to a significant extent, with more than 69 percent confirming the acquisition of knowledge from other than KHG trainers
- was effective in treatment of ailments like cold, cough, dysentery, stomach pain, white discharge, headache and fever
- was eco-system specific and listed over 106 medicinal plants and kitchen spices known for their use in home remedies
- enabled the rural resource poor to save on health expenditure, which households confirmed to be at an annual average of over Rs 1,000.

In 2000–2001, the programme was able to reach over 50,000 households, where more than a million medicinal plant saplings were planted, raised, and used for simple health care problems. In the process, it was also confirmed that the programme is self-sustainable, in the sense that the rural resource-poor members have paid more than a million rupees for the saplings planted in their kitchen gardens. It is now planned to extend the reach of the programme to cover more than a million households in the next three to five years. This will be supported by further capacity-building measures whereby any interested individual or institution would be able to implement the scheme with the help of a do-it-yourself manual on kitchen herbal gardens that is already available for use.

9

Our Living Medical Heritage[56]

Trisivaperur's Poison Specialist

Trisivaperur is the old name for Trissur—Lord Shiva's home. The combination of four words *thru, shiva, per, oor* means 'the place with Lord Shiva's name'. "*Pampu kadiyanengil atu manakkel tampurattiyude aduthu poya mati*" (If it is a snakebite, go to the *tampuratti*[57] of *mana;* that is enough.): this is what a villager, beaming with confidence, said when I asked him about the tradition of treating poisonous bites. He was referring to Vimala Antharjanam.

Vimala Antharjanam, a young housewife of Ullannor *mana* (the word *mana* means a Brahmin house) of Venkitangu *Panchayat*, started her practise as *visa vaidya* (poison specialist) soon after she got married to the second son of Ullanoor *mana*. He belonged to a Brahmin farming family. She started when she was barely 16 years old and has been practising successfully for 26 years now. She recollects how she began practising. "Once I was stepping out of the temple, and one of our family friends was coming towards the temple. He requested me to treat his son whom a dog had bitten."

This friend knew that she had been trained by her father, who was well known for his skill in treating almost all kinds of poisonous bites. He lived in one of the villages of Palakkadu in Kerala. After her marriage, Vimala Antharjanam carried the tradition of *visa vaidyam* to Trissur district.

She was drawn to this tradition from early childhood, when she started learning under her father. Her father, *Vaidya* V.M. Cherukulappurathu Shankaran Namboodiri, a famous physician, appreciated her enthusiasm. She also derived inspiration from one of her forefathers, Agnisarma, a reputed

---

[56] The subchapters 9.1-9.8 have been contributed by A. Hafeel, B.S. Somasekhar, Joel Deepak D' Silva, R. Prabha, M. Abdul Kareem, M.B. Gayatri, Sarbeswar Kar, Harish Bhat, Prabhakar Achar, Vishnu Mathur, Meera Rammohan and P.M. Unnikrishnan.

[57] Honorific title for an upper class married lady.

visa vaidya. Her interest in Sanskrit helped her in her studies since the healing traditions of Kerala, both codified and non-codified, are very strongly interrelated with, and in many cases based on, the principles of Ayurveda. The use of classical methods of diagnosis and treatment as mentioned in the *Susruta Samhita* (*Susruta*) and *Astanga hrdaya* (*Vagbhata*) is common in Kerala.

Vimala Thampuratti's family tradition dates back more than three centuries. Her father learned from Thanjavoor Krishnan Namboodiri, a descendant of Cherukulappurathu Krishnan Namboodiri, both legends in the tradition of treating snakebite. During the course of her study, along with *Upadesam* –– oral and practical teaching from the *guru* — she learned Sanskrit *kavyas* (poetry) and texts like *Astanga hrdayam, Susruta Samhita,* and *Jyotsnika, Prayogasamuccayam.* The last two texts, *Jyotsnika* and *Prayogasamuccayam*, are exclusively devoted to *visa cikitsa* (treatment of poison).

Snakebites from several species of snakes, dog bites, rodent and cat bites and poisonous bites of scorpions and spiders — she treats them all, irrespective of the stage of the condition and its severity. She says: "The incidence of snakebites increases with the monsoon and harvesting seasons, and usually the main culprits are the viper, the cobra and the krait. Curiously, it is not uncommon for people to come running with 'suspected bites' when all they need is just some comfort and some simple medication."

Her treatment involves nasal drops, orally administered medicine, eye drops and strict food regulations. Medication is based on the severity and type of poisonous bite. But the initial mixture (using the root of the plant *ottamarunnu*), which is collected from the garden, is given immediately. Strict *pathya* (diet restrictions) is always advised in the case of snakebites.

Apart from poisonous bites, she also treats skin conditions. Childcare also forms a part of her practise. It is believed that the bites' effects on the body are due to the curse of the snake; thus removing the poisonous effect from the victim will impart some of this effect onto the physician. Treating innocent children acts as a *pratikriya* (antidote) for this ill effect. "A snake bites somebody either because it mistakes him or her for prey, or when it is hurt or due to the wrongdoings of the individual in his or her past or present life."

She relates the causes of snakebites to reasons that are both tangible (and known) and intangible (and unknown).

She treats the needy without charging any fee. "People anyway are troubled with *prana* (life) and charging them adds to their troubles," Vimala Antharjanam says with a grimace, as if reprimanding all those who take advantage of the victim's helplessness. She believes greed to be a dangerous element that can ruin a good medical practise. According to her, a physician should avoid falling into this trap: "The prayers of the relieved ones give a lot more than the material gain from the treatment."

She collects most of the plant resources from her family land, which also has a couple of *kavu* (sacred groves). The treatment starts with the administration of a single drug that is grown in the garden. She also prepares and dispenses medications like *gutikas* (pills). Since *gutikas* are used in very small quantities and only for a short time, she does not prepare them frequently. These preparations involve mercury and minerals along with many other potent parts of medicinal plants, some of which have to be purchased from the market. The resources, methods of preparation and other related aspects are all in keeping with the tradition. The medications are kept secret because it is strongly felt that the patient's familiarity with the drug (in the form of a common plant) has a reduced effect. Or, as she puts it: "They never take the medicine with enough seriousness if they are very familiar with it." Psychological considerations are very important in the treatment of poisons.

The treatment also includes *duta laksana* (signs of the messenger), which involves minute physical and psychological readings of signs and symptoms. The actions and expressions of the person who brings in the patient to the *vaidya* and other external signs (sounds of lizards, falling of a dry branch, etc.) are considered important for the treatment by the *vaidya* and their significance is strictly adhered to in the diagnosis. For example, if the *vaidya* is standing anointed and preparing for his/her bath when the patient arrives, the prognosis is considered to be bad. The psychological symptoms displayed by the patient (such as hallucinations) are considered to indicate advanced stages of poisoning.

The Palakkadu tradition of *visa vaidyam* has spread to the rural areas of Trissur and serves central Kerala as well as the southern regions of Malabar. This has made the *Ullannoor mana* of Venkitangu synonymous with *visa cikitsa*. Vimala Antharjanam's courage, care and concern stand out in this area of healing. The goodwill and farsightedness of a father, combined with the zeal of a daughter, enabled this healing service to spread to other regions of Kerala. V.M.C. Namboodiri could foresee that his daughter's ability would surely benefit other parts of Kerala after she got married. She feels happy that she has been able to translate his vision into reality. Her son Brahmadathan is now completing his studies under his grandfather and is getting ready to carry forward the tradition. For the people of Trissur and Malabar this is a sign of hope.

Urdigere's Poison Specialist

His method of diagnosing an ailment is not lengthy. "We simply examine the eyes or the pulse and such like bodily symptoms." His treatment is not complicated either, though it appears unusual. Thirumalaiah, a traditional *visa vaidya*, is popularly known in the region as 'Mantrada Thirumalaiah', since the chanting of mantras is an indispensable part of his treatment. He is based at Urdigere, a small village situated 15 km east of Tumkur in Karnataka, South India.

With his seemingly simple treatment procedure that largely consists of the chanting of *mantras* and the vigorous waving of a broomstick, he has successfully treated several thousands of people for poisonous bites, skin ailments, wounds and body swellings.

Poisonous bites from snakes, vipers, scorpions, lizards, spiders and other venomous creatures; several kinds of blisters, boils, sores, open wounds, rashes, allergic reactions and other skin disorders; swelling and eruptions on the body and tissue decay — all these are common ailments for which people come to Urdigere for treatment throughout the year.

Except for those suffering from poisonous bites, the treatment strategy adopted by Thirumalaiah for all other ailments is simple and uniform. It includes the chanting of some *mantras*, followed by the administration of a drug.

However, for snakebites, he immediately administers an antidote that induces vomiting. But subsequently, these victims are also treated with the chanting of *mantras*.

The chanting of *mantras* is thus an indispensable part of all treatments. It involves the *vaidya* holding a broomstick in his right hand and waving it vigorously in a circular fashion, often touching the affected parts of the patient with the sticks, and simultaneously voicing the chants. Before he begins chanting, the *vaidya* makes it a point to turn in the direction of the local deity who is seated atop the adjacent hill. Quite surprisingly, the patients find this extremely soothing. They report that their pain recedes instantly during the course of chanting. The waving and chanting is repeated until the patient is fully relieved of the pain. In real time, the chanting of *mantras* lasts for only about two or three minutes.

The chanting is followed by the prescription of a drug. The *vaidya* dispenses a small quantity of herbal powder to all the patients. They receive it with their right palm and with great reverence. The *vaidya* ensures that every patient takes the drug in his presence. He never allows the patient to take the drug home. This powder, which is extremely bitter, is a finely ground mixture of dried leaves, roots and tubers.

Apart from the powder, which is orally administered, the *vaidya* also gives a balm to patients who have open wounds. This balm, prepared by the *vaidya* himself, comprises a small lump of butter made from cow's milk, mixed with the extracts of certain medicinal plants and raw drugs. (The *vaidya* insists that the butter be obtained only from native breeds.) The patients are advised to apply this balm and dress the wound everyday.

All the patients, irrespective of their ailment, are advised to strictly follow a diet prescribed by the *vaidya*. This consists largely of Bengal gram, rice gruel and a few selected vegetables, as well as light coffee or tea. Milk, eggs, meat, spicy and oily foods, bakery and other confectionery items are all strictly forbidden.

The treatment usually lasts for several days and often extends to a few weeks. The *vaidya* usually treats people with allergies, rashes and pains as outpatients, while those who are immobile due to poisonous bites, open wounds and tissue decay are housed in a small clinic. This clinic was recently built with support from the District Forest Department and the Foundation for Revitalisation of Local Health Traditions (FRLHT). The *vaidya* does not charge any fee; all payments are voluntary. He offers his services between 8 a.m. to 10 a.m. in the morning and 3 p.m. to 5 p.m. in the afternoon throughout the year, without any break.

The *vaidya* uses about 25 different medicinal plants and raw drugs in his treatment. Several of them are available in the forest area around the Devarayana Durga Hills, which are at a distance of about 5 km from Udigere. The remaining are obtained from a raw drug store.

Clad in a loose shirt and equally loose shorts, with a towel on his left shoulder, the *vaidya* looks like a typical farmer of the dry plains of Karnataka. He does, in fact, belong to a family of farmers. Sixty-five years old, with no formal education, he has over 40 years of experience in treating different kinds of poisonous bites. His understanding of poisonous bites, toxic substances and antidotes is quite astounding.

In spite of several thousands of successful cures and more than four decades in the profession, Thirumalaiah remains humble when it comes to the question of learning and sharing knowledge. "Knowledge is the Gods' property. Maybe I have acquired the skills of *visa vaidya* over the years, but I was not born with this knowledge. I, too, had to depend on someone while learning the basics of my profession … knowledge has to be shared for the sake of humankind…." He underlines the importance of sharing knowledge while fondly recollecting how he accidentally found his teacher. About 45 years ago, he met a sage who taught him the *mantras* and the medical plants required for treating poisonous bites.

In his effort to continue the tradition of *visa vaidya*, he has groomed a few disciples. The latest additions to this small but significant group are his two grandchildren aged 10 and 12. While expressing his concern for continuing the tradition, he emphasises that the attributes necessary for a person to be eligible are that "… the person should be interested, committed to the cause, service oriented and should never consider knowledge as the means to a livelihood. His ability to utter the *mantras* should be perfect. Finally, he should not be disturbed by human passions. Anybody fulfilling these criteria can come to me...."

He adds: "I wish I had a community herbal garden in this place from where I could distribute the required seedlings of medicinal plants to the people."

Ankola's Miracle Workers

The term 'paralysis' strikes fear in most hearts; it is also a serious concern in the medical fraternity. But in Belambar (Ankola), a family of traditional practitioners sees it as just another disease, the cure for which can be found in the plant kingdom. Bommu Shivu Ganga Gowda, winner of the FRLHT Outstanding Folk Practitioner Award for 1995, is a third-generation member of the famous Gowda family known for its special 'Ankola treatment' for paralysis.

People with paralysis come to Belambar from all over India and even abroad, especially when other types of treatment have not worked. It is the last resort for many who later realise that it should have been their first, and the first resort for others who later spread the word of the treatment that works 'a miracle'.

Belambar, 5 km from Ankola in Uttar Kannada District, is a small village untouched by urban life. It has the Sahyadri Hills to the north and the Arabian Sea to the south. People have lived in this mountainous region for 200 years, making a living from agriculture, forest produce and cattle grazing. Allopathic medicine was unknown until recently. Every sickness was dealt with using herbs, shrubs, roots, fruits, etc.

Patients are said to have come with dangling limbs and simply walk away healed after treatment. Such is the success story of this *Sanjivini* (or *Ramabana* medicine, as it is popularly known) that it is exported to London, Germany, the US, Japan, Sri Lanka and the Middle East. It is distributed in almost every state in India.

With 200 years of history behind it, this medicine has cured thousands of people, including eminent freedom fighters, politicians as well as industrialists. In 1927, the freedom movement was heading towards a decisive phase when Mahatma Gandhi was affected by a paralytic stroke. Dr Hardikar and other freedom fighters persuaded him to undergo the Belambar treatment and he did. To his surprise, he was cured within two weeks. Bommu Shivu Ganga Gowda narrates this story with pride. (Though interesting, this story has not been verified.)

Paralysis doesn't spare the mighty or the rich. According to one patient: "I was admitted to the Breach Candy hospital in Bombay for blockage of veins in the heart. We spent a few lakh rupees there without any results. Then, on someone's recommendation, I came here and I am now almost cured after being treated for 80 days and spending only Rs 300." It is claimed that many public personalities have been successfully treated here.

The Gowda tradition of healing is said to have begun when Bommu Ganga Gowda, a traditional health practitioner and cowherd, met a *sanyasi*. The *sanyasi* asked him to treat his paralysis. Bommu Ganga Gowda expressed his inability to cure it. The *sanyasi* was furious and is supposed to have asked him: "You are living in the foothills of the rich Sahyadri and are unable to treat paralysis?" Gowda told him he had not even heard of such a sickness. The *sanyasi* named a few herbs and shrubs and asked Bommu Ganga Gowda to fetch them from the forest. The *sanyasi* then explained to him how the medicine should be prepared and administered. The *sanyasi* was cured. News about his cure spread quickly and patients started coming in from other neighbouring villages.

When Bommu Ganga Gowda died, his son Shivu Bommu Ganga Gowda took over the healing tradition. It was during this period that the medicine became so popular that it was introduced into the international market. Shivu Gowda was the man who claimed to have cured Gandhi and other freedom fighters. His son recalls that his charge for treatment was a coconut, 25 paise and some betel leaves and nuts in a box.

On Shivu Gowda's death, his son Bommu Shivu Ganga Gowda took over. The 60-year-old healer is more advanced in his style of treatment than his predecessors. He first discusses the problem with the patients, examines them, and only then prescribes medicines. He has completed courses in Ayurveda and homeopathy and is well versed in modern medical theory. His diagnosis centre has no equipment, though there is a small room behind it where medicines are prepared. His clinic can now house 20 in-patients.

Bommu Gowda's family firmly believes that the names of the herbs and other ingredients that go into the preparation of the medicine should not be revealed. Commenting on the success of his method, he says: "If the patient's nervous system is active, he can be cured in two weeks; but if his nervous system is non-functional, it can take about a month or two."

The medication process is as follows: Adults are provided with a bunch of shrubs and leaves, which are divided into seven portions. Each portion is used every day for seven days. Each portion has to be ground with water and nine cloves, nine pepper pods, nine garlic pods, a half inch turmeric piece, and four spoons of mustard. This mixture is divided into two portions. One portion is kept separately, and the patient has to consume two to three spoons of it in the morning after tea. The remainder is rubbed from head to toe in a downward movement. The second portion is used in the same way, but in the evening around 4 p.m. The following morning, the patient is advised to take a hot water bath. However, it is recommended that during the first week of treatment, the patient should only cleanse the body with a wet cloth. For children, a similar method is advised but the proportion of the medicine is halved. It is important to observe silence while the medicine is being applied.

After seven days of this treatment, a face-to-toe black oil massage is administered. The oil used is mixed with numerous herbs. A woman having her periods is advised not to undergo the treatment, and men and women are both advised to remain celibate during the seven days of leaves and shrubs medication. Consumption of milk, curds, buttermilk, butter, ghee, coconut oil, sugar or jaggery, brinjal, meat and fish is banned while the treatment is ongoing.

Though three generations have been serving the people and the fourth is on the verge of taking over, the government has not recognised the service and dedication of this family. In 1967-68, when people from Sri Lanka and other countries began to use his medicine, the central government directed the Divisional Commissioner to prepare a report on Gowda's work. The commissioner recommended that since every year about 4,000 patients come to the village, provision should be made for a road, water, electricity and an indoor hospital. However, nothing was done and Bommu Gowda built his own small hospital.

He has trained many modern doctors, but none have bothered to write technical reports on his work. The plants used by him are available in the forest but they are now difficult to obtain due to the rapid deforestation occurring in these areas. Bommu Gowda would like to have some forest areas reserved for medicinal plant conservation in the Karwar region. Apart from this, he has no wishes, no dreams, no longings. He is a content man with a son who will carry on the medical tradition. He has also ensured the respect and dignity of his family name and given the world a remarkably effective treatment for what has often been considered an incurable problem.

***Nativaidya* Narayana Murthy**

Narasipura is a small village in Shimoga District of Karnataka. It is also the home of *Vaidya* Narayana Murthy.

When we visited him, he greeted us with a warm, friendly smile. A very popular figure in the area, it is not an exaggeration to say that he has become a household name in the entire district. This became evident to us while we were driving from Shimoga to the village. Wherever our vehicle stopped, we struck up small conversations with the locals. Everybody we spoke to seemed to have met or at least heard of him. On the Wednesday evening that we met him, he had some patients with him. The phone rang constantly. The *vaidya's* daughters, who assist him in his work, told us that around 600 patients had already phoned in for an appointment for the next day.

The middle-aged *vaidya* (who is basically a farmer) developed a passion for healing around 18 years ago. Healing is a legacy he has inherited from his uncle and is the family's fourth-generation *vaidya.*

He treats a wide range of ailments: cancer, kidney stones, asthma, blood sugar and heart diseases. Cancer and kidney stones, though, are his areas of specialisation. For kidney stones, the treatment he prescribes comprises a single drug for a single day. The medicines he prepares are not complex and he personally hands over the roots, bark or leaves to the patients. He also provides them with detailed information on how to prepare the medicine, the mode of administration, the dosage, the duration of treatment, and the *pathya* or diet. All the procedures are simple and often the medicinal preparation is nothing but a concentrated decoction of the drug or an extract of the drug mixed with a little honey or lime juice. His patients, who come from different socio–economic backgrounds, have great faith in his healing powers. For example, even when they can easily access the medicinal plant or its requisite part, they insist that he personally hand it over to them. The publicity-shy *vaidya* finds it difficult to adjust to the idea of handling so many patients. Nevertheless, he claims that he enjoys his work.

With no formal background in medicine, the *vaidya* has an intriguing way of treating his patients. He consults the modern diagnostic reports, which patients are required to bring along with them, and then prescribes a drug. He has a strong faith in divine intuition. He attributes his healing powers to his family deity and has built a temple dedicated to the deity very close to where he lives. He does not charge a fee for his services, though most patients do make voluntary donations, which are all passed on to the village temple.

The raw drugs he uses consist of bark, roots, and occasionally, fresh leaves. Come rain or shine, he goes out to collect the raw drugs a day prior to their dispensation. Before harvesting the plant or tree, he performs a small ritual of first circling and then prostrating himself before it. He then harvests the medicinal part. He is evasive about the total number of plant sources he uses, but he hints that they could be around 30.

On Thursdays, Narasipura village wears a very different look. The Thursday that we were there was no exception. Long winding queues of patients from different age groups and with varied medical complaints greeted us at the *vaidya's* residence. We were told that the patients were waiting there from seven o'clock in the morning. The *vaidya* begins meeting the patients from 8 a.m. onwards to beyond 4 p.m. in the evening. Except in cases of emergency, he meets patients only on Thursdays and Sundays, as these days are believed to be *Siddi vaara* or days that yield good results.

The *vaidya* took a little time off from his busy schedule to show us around his *'varada vana'*. This is the place where he collects raw drugs. He owns 25 acres of land in which grow many medicinal plant species like *Alstonia scholaris, Terminalia arjuna, Cassia fistula, Biophytum sensitivum, Pterocarpus marsupium, Rauvlfia serpentina, Plumbago zeylanica,* etc. Setting up a herbal garden where he can cultivate medicinal plants for a year-round supply of raw drugs has been a long-time dream. This project has already taken shape with some financial assistance from FRLHT and technical support from the Government Ayurvedic College, Bangalore. The Sasya Sanjivini Sangha, an NGO in Shimoga and the Karnataka Forest Department are also providing assistance for the project, which aims to cultivate over 40 different medicinal plant species.

Ten Generations of Eye Physicians

Vaidya Nagaraja Mudaliar of Olagapuram, Tamil Nadu represents an outstanding example of a family, which has been practising traditional eye medicine for the past ten generations. Village Olagapuram is situated by Kalveli tank in Vanur taluk of Villupuram district. The village is spread over 350 hectares, of which a sizeable chunk is forestland. Villagers live by collecting and selling the fruits of *Phoenix sylvestris*, *Eugenia cuminii* and *Spondias pinnata*, the flowers of *Nelumbo nucifera,* the seeds of *Azadirachta indica* and *Madhuca longifolia* and the leaves of *Agave roxburghiana* from the forest, which is also said to contain around 200 identified medicinally important plant species. The *Villi*, who are the tribal inhabitants of the village, catch snake, mongoose, rabbit and wild rats. The village also boasts of about 12 acres of sacred and temple groves and two temples — one devoted to Lord Shiva and the other to Lord Perumal. Both are of historical importance, being over a thousand years old.

Although *Vaidya* Nagaraja Mudaliar (born 1938) is primarily an eye physician, he also treats paediatrics cases, skin diseases, practices toxicology, general medicine and pre- and postoperative eye therapy. Popularly known as *Kannu Vaidyar* (eye physician), he is famous for treating cataracts using traditional methods that he traces back to his ancestors in the seventeenth century. He learnt his medical skills from his father and through the study of 48 manuscripts that were part of the family inheritance.

These palm leaf manuscripts in Tamil and Telugu cover various subjects. Six deal with the eye (*Netra Roga* and *Nidanam*), five are on childcare (*Bala graha dosa*s), 14 on general medicine, two on astrology, four on medical *mantras*, seven on *archanas*, three on diseases in general (*Gunapadam*) and seven on general medicine. With no access to proper storage and restoration facilities, however, these precious documents are now withering away.

His most precious possession, however, is his handbook, the *Netra roga nidana* written by his forefathers. This describes in great clinical detail approximately 96 *netra rogas* (eye diseases), their classifications, symptoms, diagnosis and surgical as well as non-surgical therapeutics and techniques.

Vaidya Nagaraja Mudaliar treats both surgical and non-surgical cases. Apart from the traditional skills he has acquired, he has studied books on *Peddabala sikshay* (the local language), *Nadi nidanam* (study of the pulse and its correlation with astrology to diagnose, treat and provide a prognosis), *Niti sastram* (study of behavioural patterns), *Sadrasa nighantu* (lexicon on plant drugs in different languages, i.e., Sanskrit, Telugu and Tamil), *Bhaishajya kalpa* (traditional pharmacology), *Satasloki* (eye diseases and preparation of medicines for their treatment) and *Balagraha dosa nul* (paediatrics). The last two were authored by his father, *Vaidya* Duraisamy Mudaliar.

Some important drug formulations used by *Vaidya* Nagaraja include: *Tamradi varti*, *Candrodaya varti* or *Manjal mattirai srotanjana* or *Karuppu mattirai*, *Nasika baranam sunthi* and *Ratnadi mattirai*. All these are made up of approximately 60 herbal and mineral ingredients. Although the family has the expertise to treat 96 different eye diseases, *Vaidya* Nagaraja mainly treats the following conditions:

Durmamsam

Symptoms: An external growth over the eyelid.

Procedure: The patient is made to lie comfortably on the bed with her/his eyes closed. An incision, the size of a tamarind leaflet, is made over the growth with a *sastra* (a sharp surgical instrument), which allows a white or colourless fluid to ooze out. This is cleaned and the opening is then sutured. Following fomentation with tamarind leaves, a paste of *sigru* (drumstick, *Moringa oleifera*) leaves, *tila* (*Sesamum orientale*) *taila*, onion and a pinch of turmeric (*Curcuma longa*) powder is fried and applied over the sutured area and then bandaged. The bandage is kept on for four to five days. On the sixth day, the sutures are removed and *Tamradi varti* (a medical formulation) is applied over it; and on the seventh day, *sambrani (Canarium strictum)*, turmeric and oil are heated and the paste is applied over the head. This prevents the disease from recurring.

Pattalam

Symptoms: An elongated growth over the white part of the eye (*Arma*), accompanied by redness and watering.

Treatment: In the early stages it is treated using formulations like *Tamradi varti*, *Candrodaya varti* and *Srotonjana* in equal quantities. If the growth encroaches on the black part (cornea) of the eye, it has to be treated surgically.

Pittaneer

Symptoms: Haziness of vision and inability to see objects more than 2 km away. This condition usually develops after the age of 55.

Diagnosis: A vision test is conducted by asking the patient to close one eye and recognise colours through different quadrants (fields) of the eye.

Treatment: In early stage: A combination of *Tamradi varti*, *Candrodaya varti* and *Srotanjana* is applied as *anjana* (collyrium) twice a day for five days. This is followed by *nasya* (nasal medication) with *Nasikabarana*. *Nili bhrngamalaki taila* is applied over the head for 15 days. Along with this, *Sutika* (*agnikarma*) is administered to the temporal region of the affected eye after identifying the nerves. If the patient is not able to see up to a kilometre, the treatment is extended to 10 days. Otherwise, the affliction is treated surgically.

Pre-operative procedures: If the patient has been taking a head bath daily, *Nasya* with *Nasika baranam* is given in the morning and then at night for three days. If the patient has been taking a body bath, *Candrodaya* and *Tamradi varti* are applied to the eyes as *anjana* for three days. On the fourth day, the patient has to take a head bath. Consumption of food is limited to *laghu ahara* (light diet) once a day.

Precautions: *Rahu kala* must be avoided at all costs. *Vinayaka puja* should be performed, after determining an auspicious time. Days considered suitable for operating are Tuesdays, Thursdays and Sundays.

Operative procedure: The patient has to sit facing the east while the physician has to face the south. A second person has to stand behind the patient and use his thumb to lift the upper eyelid; the physician uses his left thumb to pull open the lower eyelid. A blade-like instrument is used for this operation. The tip of the blade is tied with a thread, leaving a space the size of sesame seed (*Tila pramana*) to control its insertion. A puncture is made 1 to 1.5 mm away from the limbal region towards the temporal side. Immediately after pricking, the eyes are closed and burning charcoal is brought near the eyes to relieve pain. Later, the instrument is removed and the *salaka* (a small rod) is inserted in the incision. It is rotated gently in both a vertical and horizontal direction. This pushes the white part (lens) down. The patient is asked if he can see objects clearly. If the answer is in the affirmative, the *salaka* is removed gently. Immediately thereafter, *Tamradi varti* is applied to the operated eye.

Post-operative management: The eye is fomented with tamarind leaves. A cotton bandage, made from a square piece of clean cloth with a paste of black gram *dal* and turmeric powder applied over its four edges, is then placed over the eye. This is removed on the third day after the operation. If the eye remains red, *Tamaradi* and *Candrodaya varti* are applied as *anjana* for seven days. The patient should avoid any strain and exposure to sun, bright light, dust, wind, etc.

The same technique is found in the *Susruta Samhita, Uttra tantra*, chapter 17, where it is described as *Kaphaja linganasa* (cataract).

***Kannoi* (during the rainy season)**

Symptoms: Symptoms include swelling above the eyelids and watering, but without redness in the eyes.

Treatment: Alum (100 gm) is mixed in water (half litre), boiled and stored. Drops of this mixture are then administered to the eyes and are retained for a range of approximately 30 minutes to an hour. The eyes are then washed with hot water. Tamarind leaves are collected and ground into a *kalka* (paste). This is heated well without oil. It is then put into a *potali* (pouch) of dry cloth and applied as fomentation. A slice of lemon is taken and purified iron powder is sprinkled over it. The slice is covered with a thin white cloth and the filtered juice is squeezed over the eyes. The juice sticks to the eyes in the orbital region and turns black the next morning. A drop of the juice is applied every day to flush out the infection till the symptoms disappear.

***Kannoi* (in summer)**

***Symptoms*:** Redness of the eye, swelling, watering and discharge.

Treatment: Alum drops are administered to each eye and cotton pads are placed over them. Clean water is then poured over the eyes and the patient is made to lie down for half an hour. The pads are later replaced with a bandage of dry, cotton gauze to prevent exposure to bright light and sun.

If the problem persists, the eyes are washed with warm water the next morning. *Tamradi varti* is applied twice a day after diluting it (2 or 3 drops in each eye). *Nasyakarma* with *Nasika baranam* (nose drops) is also performed.

Kucchi padagal

Symptoms: The presence of any foreign body like a stick, sand, mud, insect, etc., in the eyes.

Treatment: The foreign body is removed. If a wound is present over the sclera, *Tamradi varti* in the form of *anjana* is applied. If it is present over the cornea, *Tamradi varti* is given in the form of drops. This treatment applies only to fresh wounds. If the patient is brought at a late stage, drops or *anjana* are not used. *Nasya karma* is given with *Nasika baranam*. This is followed by fomentation with tamarind leaves. If the swelling and watering stops but the wound still persists, *Tamradi varti* and *Candrodaya varti* are rubbed together in equal quantities and applied. If the swelling persists, *sunthi* (*Zingiber officinale*), *kasturi manjal* (*Curcuma aromatica*) and *kadukai* (*Terminalia chebula*) are rubbed in cow milk or breast milk and applied over the eyes, retained for three hours and then flushed out. This is repeated until the swelling disappears. If the patient comes to the *vaidya* at a chronic stage with a severe throbbing in the temples, *Agnikarma* (cauterisation) is performed over the eyebrows in the region exactly above the pupil.

Watering of the Eyes

Treatment: A mixture of *Tamaradi varti*, *Candrodaya varti* and *Srotanjana* in equal quantities is applied as *anjana* once a day for three to five days in the early stages.

Salesvaram

Symptoms: In this illness, the person is unable to see nearby objects clearly.

Treatment: This condition can be prevented or further deterioration can be checked with the application of *Tamradi varti* with *Candrodaya* as *anjana* or drops, twice a day for four days in a month. An oil bath with *Bhrngamalaka taila* is advisable. A paste of 15 gm each of *kadukkai* (*Terminalia chebula*), *sigru bija* (*Moringa oleifera*) and *nellikai (Phyllanthus emblica*) is mixed with the juice of lemon or *sigru* leaves or *bhrngaraja (Eclipta alba*). This is made into a *varti* and applied as *anjana* for a month. Alternately, the same paste is put in a *tamra patra* (copper vessel) and left in the sun. The drops that collect in the vessel are then applied to the eyes.

As is the fate of quite a few other local health traditions, the Olagapuram tradition also appears to be doomed after *Vaidya* Nagaraja. There is no one in the Mudaliar lineage to carry it forward. This account is thus significant for two reasons. One, it represents an exemplary case of a purely locally evolved health tradition being nurtured by a man who has charged himself with the responsibility of keeping the family tradition alive. He does this in spite of the complete lack of any institutional support, recognition or encouragement. In the process, he also provides selfless and missionary service to the community.

Two, the story of the Olagapuram tradition also represents one of numerous instances of very valuable knowledge and time-tested traditions that have proved their excellence, but are dying out due to sheer official neglect and lack of an appropriate mechanism for their preservation.

The *Pasu Vaidya* of Kadari

Kadari, an important settlement on the banks of the Kadarihole river, is situated between Mundar and Mala villages in Karkala, Karnataka. It is about 15 km from Karkala town. The western boundary of the Kudremukh National Park is about seven km from the Kadari Bridge, which marks the starting point of Mullur Ghat on the Kudremukh highway.

Srinivasa Prabhu (born 1930) is a *Pasu vaidya*, i.e., a veterinary doctor. He is well known for his work in treating a large number of cattle and sheep as well as goats and horses. He learned about animals from a very old Kannada book called *Pasu Raksa Samgraha.* Written by the late *Vaidya* M.H. Narayana Shetty (born 1910) of Higran village in Karkala Taluk, the book is a two-part compilation (*samgraha*) of 45 different veterinary ailments and their treatment as practised by the *pasu vaidyas* of Karkala taluk. Part I deals with the pathology of cattle and the procedure of cattle care. This includes the development of breed, pregnancy care, post-pregnancy care and the technique for delivery. Part II deals with the treatment of diseases.

He was very impressed with the book as it contained detailed explanation of the treatment for different veterinary diseases. With great enthusiasm he began treating his own cattle. This proved to be very successful. He then experimented with the cattle in his neighbourhood. Later, he began to treat cattle in a large number of nearby villages. He prepared his own medicines by collecting plants from the nearby forest. Since he was the Panchayat president, he travelled extensively and soon he became famous in the entire *taluk.* Since he did not charge for the treatment he provided, the poor farmers benefited tremendously.

Apart from the usual ailments, he has successfully cured some more complicated diseases as well. Based on his long and wide-ranging experience in the field, he has managed to find a cure for some diseases that were not even mentioned in the *samgraha.* The increasing demand for his services keeps him extremely busy, but he has managed to find the time to document his experience (treatment methodology) in a book, which is written in the local language. By following the instructions documented in the book, farmers can now attempt to treat their cattle on their own.

Some Examples of Disease/Treatment

Kudure kutthha roga

Symptoms: Shivering, fever, salivation and pain in legs resulting in an inability to walk. A typical sound is also heard while breathing (showing an obstruction in the respiratory tract). This disease occurs only after the beginning of the rainy season and lasts till early winter.

Treatment:

Step 1: A mixture of the leaves of *tumbe* (*Leucas indica*), *nekki* (*Vitex negundo*), *badhane* (*Solanum melongena*), *oma* (*Trachyspermum ammi*), *Sasuve* (*Brassica juncea*), *belluli* (*Allium sativum*), *sanna menasu* (*Solanum capsicum var. annum*) and *chigili* (*Rhopedelia* sp.) is ground. No water is to be added. This mixture is then wrapped in a fresh cloth and dipped in a vessel containing warm water. It is then squeezed into the nostrils of the animal.

Step 2: A handful of *bili tharoli* (*Symplocos racemosa*) leaves are ground in some water and the juice extracted. Then *adike* (*Areca catechu*) is rinsed in four to five cups of warm water. *Belluli* (*Allium sativum*), *oma* (*Trachyspermum ammi*), *sasuve* (*Brassica juncea*), pepper (*Piper nigrum*) and *ote huli* (*Artocarpus gomezianus*, subsp. *zeylanicus*) are added to the extracted juice and ground. Six cups of this juice mixed with a quarter cup of salt is then fed to the animal.

Step 3: The leaves of *kalu menasu* (*Piper nigrum*), *adike belu* (*Pothos scandens*) and *halasu* (*Artocarpus heterophyllus*) are added to porridge and given to the animal until it recovers.

Step 4: The leaves of *kare kai* (*Canthium parviflorum*), bark of *kornge* (*Trichilia cannaroides*), *kavante* (*Zanthoxylum rhesta*), *maddharsa* (*Ervatamia heyneana*), *sunthi* (*Zingiber officinale*, *karigirige* (*Vernonia anthelmntica*), *oma* (*Trachyspermum ammi*), *belluli* (*Allium sativum*) and *sasuve* (*Brassica juncea*) are ground and added to a *kasaya* (decoction) of *oma*. This is then made into three pills the size of an areca nut fruit. After being mixed with 2 gm of liquor, these pills are fed to the animal. This treatment is continued as long as the symptoms persist.

Step 5: A heated iron rod is placed on all four limbs of the animal.

Dodda roga/Mari roga

Symptoms: This is a dangerous disease as symptoms start showing only after the onset of severe internal problems. These symptoms include loss of appetite, drooping of earlobes, shivering with increase in the tension of blood vessels, nerves around the neck and the sides of the body, watering eyes and nose and lastly, loose and foul smelling motions mixed with blood. There is also a slight but persistent fever.

***Treatment*:** Great care should be taken when treating the animal, as it is already weak due to fever and loose motions. It is important to first improve its general health. In the early stages, if there are no loose motions, camphor and country liquor are mixed with a powder made from *peptluppu* and the roots of *Naregamia alata* and *Datura metel*. This is then added to three cups of porridge and fed to the animal through a tube made of bamboo. If loose motions persist even after 24 hours, then the powdered seeds of the *Terminalia chebula* are also added to the mixture. This will control the motions to a great extent. This medication should be continued even after recovery, at least in the period immediately following it, in accordance with the frequency prescribed by the *vaidya*.

Kalu kuntu roga

This disease spreads like an epidemic. An animal suffering from this disease should be isolated from the rest of the herd. Feeding other animals with the leftover food/fodder of the affected animal should be strictly avoided. Whenever this disease is noticed in a village, the head, earlobes and back of the cattle should be smeared with sesame oil. A small portion of the oil should be added to porridge and fed to the healthy animals; this will arrest/slow down the spread of the disease.

Symptoms: The animal suffers from fever, loss of appetite, dry nostrils and mouth; it does not masticate. The animal also stamps on the ground with its feet. Boils or lesions form between the hooves and on the inner surface of the mouth. In some cases, lesions also form on the udder, which burst open within 24 hours. Plenty of water also oozes out from the mouth.

Treatment: Immediately apply sesame oil on the head, back and earlobes of the animal. Grind the bark of *kurma* (botanically unidentified) with coconut milk, add 5 ml milk and a quarter proportion of sesame oil. Feed the affected cattle one to two glasses of this per day, depending on its health, for two days. The animal should be fed with dry straw/hay accompanied by warm porridge or liquid fodder to which 5 gm of salt has been added. Sesame oil should be given regularly. If they burst, the lesions should be smeared with camphor oil to keep the flies away.

Korallu roga

Symptoms: Its symptoms include loss of appetite, drooping earlobes, swelling in the throat, difficulty in breathing, and foaming at the mouth. There is also a progressive swelling of the neck. The affected animal should be isolated from the healthy ones.

Treatment: The animal should be given 10–15 gm of *jhadane uppu* (botanically unidentified) mixed in warm water. The swelling around the neck should be treated by applying a hot, iron rod to mark the sign '=' on either side of the neck. Its mouth needs to be washed with warm water mixed with a little tamarind. If there is any improvement, 2–3 gm of salt, 11gm of *Solanum capsicum var. suffruticosum*, 11 gm of ginger and 1 gm if chillies are powdered along with jagerry and made into pills. Two of these pills should be given to the animal twice (morning and evening) a day for three days.

Traditional Bonesetting

The Puthur bonesetting hospital lies about 20 km south of Tirupathi, towards the Tamil Nadu border. The pavement outside the hospital is strewn with small shops selling various articles — from eggs to cotton material. The customers are generally patients visiting the hospital; they are required to buy these items as the doctors in the hospital use them for treatment.

The hospital itself is a medium-sized, concrete building set in rustic surroundings. One can usually find numerous patients strolling around outside, wearing bandages or splints on various parts of their body. Entry into the hospital itself is quite an informal affair, with only a few rules for admission. The entrance is always filled with long queues of patients of all ages — some in great pain due to recent injuries, many with recent fractures that require immediate attention, and others who are there for a routine bandaging session or a second check-up. They are divided into batches of 10 and the most urgent cases are seen first.

Most of the patients are from nearby or outlying villages around the Puthur area. However, a large number of them also come from other states. One can view this as a testament to people's faith in the Puthur bonesetters. It is obvious that many come here because they are dissatisfied with treatment given by other orthopaedic units, which include some well-known modern centres.

The fee for treatment depends on what the patient can afford to pay (usually Rs 5–10 per session) and the bandages and medicines cost another Rs 5. The treatment procedure is extremely fast and efficient — so fast that it needs to be seen to be believed. On an average, the Puthur bonesetters treat about 300 patients a day!

The main ward consists of a long and fairly bare hall with 10 long wooden tables arranged alongside each other. These are a few feet apart. There is no privacy, but this does not seem to bother anyone. On an average, each patient needs about five to ten minutes for treatment. A few complicated cases, however, require more time.

The history behind this hospital is an interesting one. Gopal Raju, who lived at the turn of the century (and is the grandfather of the present chief bonesetter, Markandeya Raju), stumbled upon the discovery that certain leaves or herbs growing in the field possessed some sort of medicinal or healing properties. The story is that once, when Gopal Raju was hunting in the forest, he returned with an injured animal resting on a bed of leaves.

When he reached home, Gopal Raju found that some of the broken limbs of the animal had joined up of their own accord. He realised that the leaves were responsible for the healing. Gopal Raju decided to experiment further and tried healing the broken limbs of chickens, dogs and so forth, and found that the treatment worked for all of them. He then began using his knowledge to treat his neighbours, especially those who had fractures or other injuries. When he died, he passed this knowledge on to his sons. Since then, four generations have practised this skill, which is passed down orally or by demonstration and experience.

Markendeya Raju fears that this knowledge is likely to be exploited by those who practise bonesetting for commercial benefit. He feels that only total dedication and a sense of service on the part of the practitioner can make him/

her a good healer. Sharing this knowledge and skill to increase the number of practitioners might not necessarily increase the number of people it could benefit.

This very conviction, however, has kept Markendaya Raju from developing any sort of theoretical framework for his treatment. There has been no effort at any research into the system; nor is there any extensive written material available. But there is one important bit of modern technology that Markandeya Raju is open to and has in fact adopted: the use of X-rays. He studies the X-rays brought in by patients for diagnoses — something that he has also trained his sons to do.

Often, patients are accompanied by relatives or friends and, if necessary, carried in and placed on one of the long tables. The patients are then held still, while the bonesetter feels the actual site carefully and assesses the nature of the injury by running his hands over the area and probing with his fingers. When he finds the place and is satisfied that it is an actual fracture or dislocation, he asks for the patients to be held more firmly while he proceeds to actually 'set' the bone. He does this in the same way an orthopaedic surgeon would, by means of pushing, pulling or manipulating the fractured area in such a way that it quickly clicks back into the correct position. It is largely this procedure that showcases the skill and expertise of the bonesetter: the better a bone is 'set' the faster will be the healing process. While in an orthopaedic clinic, this procedure would be carried out under anaesthesia and strictly controlled conditions, in this hospital everything, apart from the intense concentration of the bonesetter, is very relaxed, almost casual.

After the bone is 'set', a mixture of ground leaves (or herbs) and turmeric is applied as a sort of ointment around the area of injury. It is then firmly bandaged with a piece of cotton cloth smeared with raw eggs.

The Puthur bonesetters have mastered their skill over generations. Their success is evident in the number of patients they treat everyday; their value lies in the efficient and affordable treatment they provide to those who cannot travel long distances or pay high fees for modern orthopaedic help.

Mental Health Care in a Village Setting

Poomkutil *mana* is the Namboothiri family's centre for curing mental diseases.

It presents an excellent model of community living, which is seen as essential for the treatment and rehabilitation of psychiatric patients. Situated on a three-acre plot in Vallikkappatta village (Malappuram), near the Palakkad–Manjeri state highway, Poomkutil *mana* can accommodate nearly 40 patients at a time, with about 80–100 coming in everyday as outpatients. Inpatients are accommodated in rooms around the *nalukettu* (inner courtyard).

Mental health traditions in India — both local and classical — cover a variety of practises. They include healing traditions connected with religious places such as temples and mosques, and are peopled by such practitioners as *vaidyas*, *hakims*, *siddhars*, *tantric healers*, *sadhus* and *sufis*.

Manasika roga (afflictions of mind) fall under a specialisation named *Kaya cikitsa* (general medicine) in Ayurveda, which has another branch called *Graha cikitsa* that deals with the multiple manifestations of the mind. Though both broadly follow the classical Ayurvedic tradition, we can see that the methodologies of diagnosis and treatment gradually diluted.

There is no evidence that clearly pinpoints when this tradition of Poomkutil *mana* began, though it is clearly more than 600 years old. Oral in nature, it is said that in this tradition physicians are born, not made. Each generation of the family is exposed to various aspects of mental health through everyday interactions with patients and their physician fathers. Knowledge is thus transmitted from generation to generation. At present, it is practised by a team of five physicians, all belonging to the same family — Vishnu Namboothiri, P.N. Namboothiri, Devan Namboothiri, Jathavedan Namboothiri and Narayanan Namboothiri. Although their formal education has been in different subjects, they have dedicated their lives to the practice of this art.

The treatment offered in this centre is of a very special nature. Daily special *pujas* for the family deities Ganapathy and Bhagavathy, the chanting of *mantras* along with medical treatment using methods like *sneha pana* (unction), *virecana* (purgation), *dhara* (pouring of decoction on the head and body), *nasya* (nasal medication) — are all part of the therapeutic armamentarium. It is a combination of all three modalities of treatment mentioned in the Ayurveda, i.e., *Daivavyapasraya* (spiritual therapy), *Satvavajaya* (psychological) and *Yuktivyapasraya* (rational therapy).

Daivavyapasraya consists of the recitation of *mantras*, the wearing of gems and roots, offerings and gifts to the gods and priests, the practice of religious precepts, atonement, fasting, invoking blessings, praying, pilgrimage, etc. *Satvavajaya* is the restraining of the mind from unwholesome mental activity, while *Yuktivyapasraya* consists of the rational administration of diet and drugs. Even though the physicians do not follow these Ayurvedic classifications exactly as described in Ayurvedic texts, it is evident that their treatment includes all three.

According to these physicians, successful treatment comprises four essential factors: *sneha* (love), *ausadha* (medicine), *paradevata* (family deity) and *samuham* (society), which parallel the Ayurvedic *Catuspada* (the four essentials in Ayurveda)—the physician, medicine, attendant and patient. All four factors, both in Ayurveda and according to the Namboothiri physicians, are equally important.

In this tradition, 'society' is given a lot of weightage, for it is 'society' that first diagnoses cases and brings the patients to the physicians. The physicians are careful to note even the most casual of descriptions provided by persons accompanying the patient. They believe that society has its own classification of such illnesses and that it distinguishes degrees of each illness with a local name. This is considered very important. Often, it is determined that a specific event is the cause of the illness; consequently, the physicians examine it very carefully. 'Society' is considered to play a major role even during rehabilitation, which is why the physicians try to avoid inpatient treatment as much as possible. Rehabilitation of outpatients is said to take place naturally.

The physicians consider three major factors in the diagnosis and treatment of mental diseases:

- the relationship between the mind and the external world, i.e., how changes in nature influence the mental status of an individual. For example, patients with chronic illness show variations in symptoms depending on lunar changes
- the relationship between mind and body, i.e., how disharmony in the body is reflected in the mind and vice versa

- the relationship between materials and the mind, i.e., how medicines/food affect the mind.

Based on their practical experience, the physicians have developed a number of diagnostic guidelines. For example, if patients keep repeating the same movement or the same phrases in their speech, it is considered to denote a chronic condition (in Ayurveda, this is *vata avastha* or the chronic stage). According to the physicians, when it reaches this stage, the disease would have already had a history of a minimum of three years and would thus be quite difficult to cure. Another observation is that recurring diseases respond to treatment temporarily but cannot be completely cured (according to Ayruveda, such diseases are classified under *yapya vyadhi* or diseases that can be controlled but not completely cured). There can be variations in the person affected during different time periods, and in some chronic cases (psychoses, schizophrenia, etc.) there can be fluctuations in the symptoms displayed by the patient as, for example, during the cusps of the full moon or the black moon (when the moon is not visible).

Dr Raghuram, a leading psychiatrist in the area, was asked for his views on the treatment at Poomkutil *mana*. According to him, there are very peculiar disease presentations in Malappuram district where this centre is situated. The young of this area often migrate to the Gulf for jobs. The result is that their children often lack parental care and end up with mental afflictions. The individuals who migrate suffer from diseases like paranoid psychosis (delusion or beliefs based on incorrect inferences about external reality), anxiety (persistent excessive and unrealistic worry combined with mental tension, impaired concentration and insomnia) and depression (depressed mood on a daily basis for more than two weeks, accompanied by emotions like sadness, indifference, irritation, etc).

He cited Poomkutil *mana* as an excellent example of community therapy; the centre is like a commune where patients, their family members and the physicians interact constantly and freely. Further, the treatment here can contribute substantially to tackling chronic diseases, such as manic psychosis, schizophrenia, neurosis, anxiety and depression. The drugs used by the physicians here have minimum side effects and therefore can be used for longer periods in chronic cases. *Pathya* (the dietary and daily regimen) also plays an important role in such cases. Dr Raghuram suggested the setting up of a common platform where physicians from different medical schools can combine their efforts to treat chronic problems. However, he did point out that the methods used by the centre for physically restraining patients could do with some modification.

Each year in February the centre holds a festival celebrating the *mana*'s deity, to which people from Vallikkapatta and other neighbouring villages are invited. At this time, the centre also holds a seminar on mental health, which is attended by a large number of Ayurvedic physicians, psychiatrists, and academicians. There have been a few proposals for expanding the centre, but the physicians fear that such an expansion would lead to commercialisation of the services offered. However, they are quite willing to impart their knowledge to new graduates, albeit on the condition that the students are ready to learn in the existent environment of the centre. Dr A. P. Raman, a graduate of Ayurveda College, Coimbatore, was trained here for three years and is now running the Bodhi Mental Health Centre at Coimbatore. He is also involved in a project treating persons affected by cerebral palsy and retardation.

It is encouraging to note that the children of the Namboothiri physicians of Poomkutil *mana* are already involved in helping out their parents and plan to continue this tradition in the future.

SECTION III
The Way Forward

SECTION III

The Way Forward

Epilogue

Darshan Shankar

Most people who are out of touch with the indigenous express scepticism regarding the relevance of traditional forms of knowledge, which they tend to dismiss as obsolete, limited or incomplete. If this is indeed the case, then traditional knowledge should give way to modern understandings. It is, however, very important to establish this fact before we discard traditional knowledge.

It is not uncommon for members of the 'formally educated' class to propose 'scientific' evidence for traditional knowledge. They do so without being aware of the epistemological complexities involved in the proposal. In fact, so far there has been no real attempt to make a serious and comprehensive scientific study of the Indian medical heritage. It is also true that to develop an acceptable intercultural methodology for such a study would not be an easy task, as it would need a great deal of cross-cultural insight and understanding of the paradigms of two vastly different knowledge systems. The truth of the matter is that, at present, the scientific community has little understanding of the epistemology of indigenous medical knowledge and therefore is not in a position to make any reliable judgements about the validity of its propositions.

The term 'traditional' knowledge does imply a connection with the past. It is, however, necessary to reflect on the nature of such traditions and the reasons for their continuity and wide social acceptance. It is unlikely that these long-standing traditions have remained static and unchanging over centuries, and that generation after generation has held on to them and passed them on merely out of stubbornness or blind respect for traditions perse. It is more likely that living traditions, particularly in a field such as medicine and health care, have been found to be of relevance, or else they would have been discarded long ago. Merely because the past is involved there is no reason to assume that traditional knowledge is static, unchanging or obsolete; its longevity may well be a sign of its robustness, its adaptability and of the sound principles that underlie it.

While inter- and cross-cultural medical studies hold very exciting prospects for the future of world medicine and need to be encouraged, it would be very wrong for governments to suspend, in the meanwhile, support to the indigenous medical systems of the world merely because they have not yet been understood by Western biomedicine. Given the extremely small proportion of national and international health budgets that is allocated to 'traditional systems of medicine', it appears that they have been more or less 'suspended' by official systems of governance. It is the ordinary people in India and other developing countries, and now even in Western countries, that are the biggest supporters of the traditional and complementary systems of medicine. Which is why thousands of folk healers, traditional clinics, nursing homes and complementary medicine functionaries continue to exist in various countries despite the lack of government support.

Globally, the prospects of traditional medicine have begun to look brighter than they did a few decades ago due to the resurgence of public support for complementary medicine. Governments are beginning to take note of the public expressions of support, and the present trend is towards making higher public investment.

The largest and most important challenge that practitioners and theoreticians of indigenous medicine face is therefore the revitalisation of the epistemological foundations of traditional medical knowledge systems. In India, the traditional systems of medicine have yielded thus far an 'ocean of knowledge', based on their own epistemology. This abundance of knowledge is a proof of their tremendous creativity and productivity and can be seen in terms of the large number of medical manuscripts, the vast and deep knowledge of plants, animals, metals and minerals, the thousands of formulations documented in the *materia medicas*, the sophisticated methods of processing natural materials, the schemes and techniques for diagnosis, the unique systems of treatment (e.g., p*anca karma*), the rules for healthy living, the depth of understanding of the nervous system and the mind, the science of acupressure (*Marmam*), and such writings as those of Patanjali on the *yoga sutras*. Given this impressive track record, it seems logical to assume that the creativity of indigenous knowledge can only be restored when its epistemology, which has been in limbo for the last century or so, is reactivated: today's practitioners are only living off past achievements without substantially making any new contributions.

As with indigenous systems of medicine in other nations, the biggest threat to the Indian medical heritage comes from its cooption by Western biomedicine. For instance, researchers of Indian systems of medicine (ISM) are asked to explain their drugs, therapies and concepts based on Western biomedicine parameters and the results achieved are applauded as high science and praised. Translating *slokas* to science is suggested as the way for ISM to move ahead. While collaboration with Western biomedicine is desirable, the scope, purpose and limitations of the collaboration need to be clearly understood. Collaborative projects should aim to open channels for dialogue and communication and foster mutual understanding and respect across medical knowledge systems. They cannot be seen as the means for validation, nor can they restore the basic creativity of indigenous knowledge systems.

The situation that ISM currently finds itself in, presents a complex picture. Around the world there is a surge in interest in those aspects of our heritage that can answer the health needs of rich societies. Treatments for arthritis, obesity, diabetes, diseases of old age, cardiology, skin disorders, immune deficiency, yoga for mental health and so on are much in demand. A small troop of doctors trained in traditional medicine have, therefore, found permanent shelter in the West. This foreign interest has inspired a matching response from our own urban middle and upper classes and an emerging domestic market is being created in Indian urban centres. Policymakers have also become aware of the growing size of the global herbal market and are therefore keen to ensure that India gets a reasonable share of this market. Funds for collaborative research on traditional medicine that will generate 'scientific' evidence of its efficacy have therefore started to flow in, although, unfortunately, no funds are as yet being invested to strengthen the roots and theoretical foundations of the Indian medical heritage, or to strengthen 'local health cultures' in rural areas.

The rural scene is tragic. In order to open up rural markets for their products, Western companies have needed to replace traditional beliefs and practices, which they have done by denigrating traditional medicine as obsolete and irrational. The government health services — manned by doctors trained in Western medicine — also have been inadvertently used to promote the campaign for displacing traditional medicine. Thus a section of the rural people in all social classes, including the poor, are giving up traditional health practices and turning to Western medicine. For the rural poor, this replacement of tradition has serious economic consequences and socio-economic surveys indicate that the single and largest cause of rural indebtedness is health expenditure.[58]

The situation may worsen in a few years because of the new international trade and patents regime under the World Trade Organisation. Modern pharmaceutical products are expected to become much more expensive than at present. For the average Indian citizen, and particularly for the rural and urban poor, it is likely that both modern drugs as well as manufactured and packaged traditional herbal medicines will be out of reach. Ensuring the health security of the average citizen — threatened due to market trends — will therefore be a big challenge. One, and perhaps the most viable way to insulate village communities and millions of rural and urban households from the emerging compulsions of the marketplace would be to revitalise folk medicine and household health traditions.

In the meanwhile, wild plants and other natural resources used by traditional medicine unfortunately are being eroded due to the loss and degradation of their natural habitats or over-harvesting for commercial purposes. Urgent measures for conserving wild genetic resources, as well as for kick-starting large-scale cultivation, are therefore necessary.

Wild animal parts used in ISM are no longer available, since access to them would involve killing the animal. There is an outright ban on this under conservation laws. For other animal products like musk and semen (of the civet cat) or the bile of the cow, that do not necessarily involve destruction, there were feeble, low-key attempts to experiment with captive breeding and methods of non-destructive harvesting in the 1970s, but these, too, have been suspended.

---

[58] Approach Paper to the Tenth Five-Year Plan of the Government of India, published by the Planning Commission in 2001.

In the case of metals and minerals, no assessment has been made either to determine the status of the natural resource base or to identify sustainable methods for accessing these resources. This is a totally dark area. With respect to plants (which are the most abundantly used natural resource), there have been recent initiatives for systematic, in situ conservation that will also aid the cultivation of medicinal plants by way of conserving germ plasma, which is essential for the breeding and selection of plant varieties.

In the context of medicinal plants, the most effective way to conserve inter- and intra-specific diversity would be to create a network of in situ forest reserves across the different forest habitats that exist in the country. The size of each forest reserve could be around 200 to 500 hectare in tropical areas, but may be smaller in higher altitude forests. A network of such forest reserves would serve as a gene bank for medicinal plants and provide breeders and growers access to wild genetic resources. This is a novel and cheapest method for conserving the gene pool of the country's medicinal plants. Based on it, forest departments in Peninsular India are spearheading a pioneering medicinal plants programme for in situ conservation of medicinal plants.

Ironically, while traditional systems of medical knowledge are generally eroding in their centres of origin, the issue of protecting the intellectual property rights (IPRs) of tribal, rural and traditional communities has come to centre stage the world over. International agreements like the Convention on Biodiversity (CBD) have been forged to grant 'fair terms for access to local biological resources and indigenous knowledge', and while national governments have not yet bothered to design effective strategies to revitalise indigenous medical knowledge and restore its creativity, they are making feverish attempts to protect traditional knowledge from 'patent thefts'. The Indian government has legislated a biodiversity bill and has also launched a project to computerise traditional herbal formulations and create a 'traditional knowledge digital library' that will be provided to patent offices worldwide in order to establish prior art and thus prevent false patent claims. However, some basic issues relating to IPRs and traditional knowledge are being ignored. These are:

- A piece of traditional knowledge may be 'modified' and a patent claimed on the modification by asserting that the 'modification' is novel and new.

Such modification cannot be 'prevented' merely by digitising traditional knowledge. But according to the CBD, the owners of the particular piece of traditional knowledge can seek benefit-sharing from the commercialisation of the modification, provided that commercial users are obliged to seek 'informed consent' for the use of that traditional knowledge. The problem is that much of the codified medical knowledge is already accessible because it is available as published texts or manuscripts in the major libraries of the world. Oral or uncodified knowledge is also being documented and once this happens it, too, will enter the 'public domain'.

- A more serious problem is that the present IPR regime is based on only one knowledge system: the Western. Any innovation carried out in an indigenous, non-Western knowledge system will not be recognised by the patent offices as an innovation, because evaluation of patent claims is based only on Western knowledge systems. This mono-cultural knowledge domination of the IPR regime needs to be challenged.
- Another fundamental problem stems from the philosophy of the IPR regime, which is again based on Western ethics and values. Questions are being raised as to why IPRs should be awarded only on the basis of Western ethics and values. According to the customary laws of traditional cultures, an individual or community's intellectual contributions are translated, recognised and awarded very differently.
- Further problems relate to disputes between traditional knowledge and modern knowledge. Such disputes may arise over the novelty of the modifications carried out on a piece of traditional knowledge. What may be non-obvious and novel in Western culture may be very obvious and commonplace in a traditional culture. Intercultural councils are needed to settle such disputes, but as of today there is no provision for the involvement of persons from non-Western knowledge systems in dispute settlement councils.
- Questions also arise from the political relationship between traditional knowledge and Western knowledge. A large part of the debate assumes the superiority Western knowledge systems, and looks upon 'backward' non-Western traditional knowledge systems as a source for providing 'leads' or raw materials, which can then be refined by a superior Western

knowledge system to make innovations possible. This political relationship between the knowledge systems needs to be challenged. Traditional knowledge systems are profound in their own context and can be best understood and appreciated within their own epistemological framework. While there is scope for meaningful collaborative research across medical cultures, protocols and guidelines for mutually respectful and epistemologically sensitive research have yet to be developed.

The crafting of a national agenda for the revitalisation of the Indian medical heritage that enjoys the support of society, policymakers and industry is a difficult exercise. A great deal of balancing is needed to address five major national concerns:

1 the concerns of ISM scholars regarding the neglect of the theoretical foundations of ISM and, consequently, the lack of creativity in the traditional medicine community
2 the concerns of social activists about the extremely limited contribution of ISM, both from its codified and folk streams, to public health in India, in spite of the vast numbers of practitioners and the wealth of traditional systems of health care
3 growing global interest in medical pluralism, expressed in the form of the complementary and alternative medicine movement, and the role that the ISM can play in shaping this global wave
4 the aspirations of the Indian herbal industry for becoming a world player
5 the concerns of Western biomedicine professionals and policymakers about the strategy for the popularising of Indian systems of medicine in the West by generating scientific evidence for ISM claims.

In the following section, we have outlined a 13-point revitalisation agenda that tries to address all these contemporary challenges faced by India.

Outline of a Future Agenda for the Revitalisation of the Indian Medical Heritage

Revitalisation of household health traditions

In terms of numbers, the largest and most visible users of Indian medical systems are the millions of rural and urban households. They use these in the form of preventive measures and promotional practices — which is reflected in their home remedies, health related customs, seasonal diets, etc. Since such health practices have been passed on as traditions, their rationale and logic may become obscured when they are not understood by the new generation. The likelihood of this happening increases by several times when one considers the limitations of the current formal education system that does not teach *any* indigenous science. The value of indigenous health practices is thus not appreciated and, in the process, some sound practices are lost. A number of traditional health practices are being discarded due to ignorance regarding their real value.

Since the use of such traditions by households can contribute to self-reliance in primary health care for millions, their revival through in-depth documentation, assessment and promotion should be the top priority of any revitalisation agenda. The strategy for revitalising such traditions will need a special understanding of the informal, 'people-to-people' processes of knowledge transmission that have passed on these traditions for centuries.

Revitalisation of folk health traditions

Folk health traditions are evidence of the great, decentralised people's health culture of India. The revitalisation of health traditions relating to birth attendants, herbal healers, bonesetters, *visa* healers, etc., should figure high on our agenda because folk health practitioners cater to millions of villages in the context of primary health care. Their services are both affordable and easy to access. The revitalisation of folk health traditions will need a special understanding of the oral transmission methods that have kept these traditions alive.

Collaborative research with Western biomedicine

This is an important area for codified Indian medical knowledge systems. Convincing Western medical sciences about the validity of ISMs can attract technological and financial resources that could be gainfully used in the revitalisation agenda. Collaborative research with Western biomedicine should, however, focus on those health problems that have inadequate or no solutions in Western medicine. Only this kind of research will have any useful impact. It is possible that research may yield more efficacious and cheaper treatments and there may well be spin-offs in identifying novel modes of action. Pulse diagnosis (*Nadi pariksa*), acupressure (*Marma vijnana*) and pharmacy (*Bhaisaja kalpana* and *Rasa sastra*) are other unexplored areas that hold promise. It would also be useful to make a serious effort to include selected traditional Indian herbal formulations in the pharmacopoeias of modern medicines.

Predictive medicine is a new branch of medicine that is beginning to evolve. It seeks to predict health problems that an individual or community is likely to face based on genetic make-up, diet, geographical location and so on. The Ayurvedic concept of *prakrti*, combined with genetics, holds exciting prospects for collaborative research.

Conservation and use of medical manuscripts

Manuscripts form a reliable source of authentic traditional medical knowledge. Unfortunately, they often lie neglected and many are now lost. Cataloguing the vast number of medical manuscripts, conserving and publishing critical editions — are all a vital part of the revitalisation agenda. Monographs need to be prepared in speciality areas like *Netra cikitsa* (opthalmology), *Marma* and *Varmam cikitsa* (acupressure and orthopaedics), *Danta cikitsa* (dentistry), *Prasuti tantra* (maternity care), *Manasika roga* (mental diseases), *Visa cikitsa* (treatment of poisons). Although this area of work may not deliver immediate benefits, it is crucial for long-term sustenance.

Restoring creativity in educational institutions

Another crucial area for urgent action is undergraduate, post-graduate and in-service refresher education in ISM. The poor quality of education has had a crippling effect on India's medical heritage. Current education programmes are weak in design, structure, methods and infrastructure, generating a cadre of deficient practitioners and researchers who will not be able to serve the revitalisation agenda. The growing demand for ISM courses in foreign countries is one more reason why traditional medical education in India needs to be strengthened. In this context, an important point to remember is that whilst using modern languages for communication, it is vital to continue to use Sanskrit, Tamil and Persian for teaching the core of the subject because the depth and clarity of the language and the uniqueness of concepts would be difficult to translate into other languages.

Support research on the epistemology of ISM

In the last century, indigenous knowledge systems have experienced serious stagnation. Foundational research on their epistemology can help rediscover the operational methodology of ISM and thus reactivate traditional knowledge systems and restore their creativity so that they can become self-generating again. This is a fundamental area in any revitalisation agenda and needs active and substantial policy support.

Clinical research based on ISM parameters

Clinical research based on ISM parameters and protocols can help to restore self-confidence in young ISM clinicians by demonstrating the validity of their own knowledge systems. Since ISM clinics all over India are the largest instrument for ISM practice, it is essential to include clinical research in any revitalisation agenda for Indian systems of medicine. The focus of clinical research should be on the most important public health priorities.

Medical pluralism

'Bridging research' is intended to correlate the fundamental concepts of different medical traditions. A basic knowledge of principles and treatment norms of ISM should be introduced into the curricula for modern medicine and vice versa. This research will help in the design of courses on complementary and alternative medicine that are now being slowly introduced in medical curricula in India and abroad.

Application of information technology (IT)

The application of IT to organise traditional medical knowledge can lead to its more efficient utilisation in teaching, clinical practice and research. It is important to use this new tool to strengthen the applications of Indian systems of medicine. The areas of application include databases on *materia medicas*, diagnostics, special therapies (like *Pancakarma* and *yoga*) and specialty fields (orthopaedics, pharmacy ophthalmology, paediatrics, *Rasayana* therapies, etc.). It could also be effectively used for the protection of IPRs relating to traditional knowledge.

Conservation of medicinal plants and other natural resources

Conservation of wild populations of medicinal plants in their natural habitats will ensure their long-term availability. The supply of germ plasma and botanically authentic planting materials will be also ensured. Additionally, trade in endangered species collected from the wild needs to be regulated.

The promotion of organic cultivation strategies based on the principles of '*desa vicara*' can ensure the availability of raw materials to user groups. Also, it can provide income and employment to small, marginal farmers and rural women. Apart from plants, it is equally necessary to develop programmes for the conservation and sustainable utilisation of animal resources, metals and minerals.

Herbal products for domestic use and export

Apart from Indians in both rural and urban areas, there is also an emerging market for ISM products in Europe, USA, Japan, Australia, Russia, Africa and South America. A balanced strategy is therefore needed to meet domestic and global consumer demands. Competent clinical and manufacturing practices and standards related to cultivation thus require to be evolved. In this context, care should be taken that such standards are not imposed arbitrarily. Care should also be taken to ensure that modern technology is used only to delineate and build upon the traditional standards of ISM. Since the quality of raw material used is of great importance, research should be directed towards establishing simple methods for quality control that could be followed even at the local level.

International cooperation

Historically, Indian medical traditions have had a strong influence on the development and practice of medicine in various parts of South East Asia, particularly China, Thailand, Vietnam, Burma, Indonesia, Sri Lanka and Nepal. Chinese travellers who visited the great Indian universities at Nalanda have reported the presence of a large number of students from outside India studying a variety of subjects, including medicine. Since their medical traditions have a lot in common with the medical traditions of India, this is an important role that we should continue to play through interaction with other countries in region that are trying to revive their own traditional health practices.

Traditional agricultural and veterinary sciences

It is interesting and fascinating to see that the Indian medical heritage is not restricted to the treatment of human beings. There are two other facets, of which one is the practice of *Mrgayurveda* or traditional veterinary medicine. We have not only a large number of manuscripts on this subject but also a number of traditional practitioners who may be called 'ethno-veterinary practitioners'. Some of these practitioners have outstanding abilities and experience.

Similarly, there are a large number of manuscripts as well as farming practices pertaining to the area of *Vrksayurveda*, i.e., traditional plant science. This second facet covers varied aspects of horticulture like soil testing, selection and storage of seeds, nursery techniques and plant propagation methods, use of manures and fertilizers, irrigation, pest control and disease management, and the recognition of favourable meteorological conditions for agricultural operations.

These two areas represent a body of knowledge and information that can be explored, strengthened and built upon.

Conclusion

Given the current global and domestic trends, it seems that the 'time' for executing a well-conceived revitalisation strategy for the Indian medical heritage has come. It is also obvious that in order to execute such a strategy, we would need to enlist a large measure of domestic and international cooperation. There are several paths that can be taken, but not all of them will result in the revitalisation of India's medical heritage. It is our hope that this book will light up pathways that will be the most appropriate for the revival of the indigenous medical heritage of India.

About the Editors

Darshan Shankar

Darshan Shankar began his professional work in 1973 at the University of Bombay, where he conceived, designed and coordinated (1973–80) a postgraduate 'experiential learning programme'. This programme offered two-year fellowships to graduates of different disciplines to live in rural areas and develop socially useful action–research projects. In 1976, the programme received a Commonwealth Award after being adjudged the best project in the Commonwealth for linking university education to community needs.

Between 1980 and1992, Shankar lived in a tribal area in Maharashtra, where he worked with a grassroots, non-government organisation called the Academy of Development Science. It was during this period that he was exposed to the tremendous social relevance of local health traditions.

Since 1993, Darshan Shankar has been the Director of the Foundation for Revitalisation of Local Health Traditions (FRLHT), Bangalore. In 1998, he received the Norman Borlaug award and in 2002, the medicinal plant conservation programme in peninsular India, coordinated by FRLHT, received the United Nations' Equator Initiative Prize.

Email – darshan.shankar@frlht.org.in

P.M. Unnikrishnan

Unnikrishnan studied at the Ayurveda College, Coimbatore and graduated as an Ayurvedic physician in 1992. In the same year, he founded (with some friends) the Centre for Ayurvedic Research and Development (CARD), a network of clinical centres in Kerala to promote classical Ayurvedic practice and research. After graduation, he worked as a Research Fellow at the famous Amala Cancer Hospital and Research Centre in Kerala, and was also a Visiting Research Fellow at the Toyama Medical and Pharmaceutical University, Toyama, Japan.

Although Unnikrishnan completed his post-graduation in Medical Anthropology at the University of Amsterdam in 2000, he has been working with the Foundation for Revitalisation of Local Health Traditions from 1995. He spent his initial years at FRLHT building up a database of medicinal plants used in Ayurveda. He is currently coordinating the Traditional Systems of Medicine (TSM) unit of the Foundation. His professional interests include cross-cultural medical research, relevance of traditional medicine in public health and applied medical anthropological research.

Email – unni.pm@frlht.org.in

About the Authors

A. V. Balasubramaniam obtained his MSc degree in Chemistry from Bangalore University and a post-MSc diploma in Molecular Biophysics from the Indian Institute of Science, Bangalore. He later studied Physiology and Biophysics at the State University of New York at Stonybrook. From 1982 onwards, his work centred around exploring the current relevance and potential of Traditional Indian Sciences and Technologies, with special emphasis on Yoga and Ayurveda. In 1986, he joined the Lok Swasthya Parampara Samithi (LSPSS) as Editor of Publications. He is currently the Director of Centre for Indian Knowledge Systems, an institution devoted to exploring the contemporary relevance and applications of Indian Knowledge Systems.

A. Hafeel graduated in Ayurveda from the Ayurveda College, Coimbatore in 1998, when he joined the Foundation for Revitalization of Local Health Traditions (FRLHT) as Programme Officer in charge of coordinating the Documentation and Rapid Assessment of Local Health Traditions (DRALHT) project. His professional interests include developing and promoting appropriate methodologies for bridging various medical sciences in the context of primary health care.

G. Hariramamurthy is a Senior Programme Officer in the Exsitu Conservation Unit of the Foundation for Revitalization of Local Health Traditions. As a Task Force Leader of Kitchen Herbal Garden Programme, he is currently coordinating the implementation of Community Participation Programmes through the Medicinal Plants Conservation Parks in the states of Karnataka, Kerala and Tamil Nadu. He is alsothe HonoraryConvenor of Medicinal Plants Conservation Network and a founder-member of the Paramparika Vaidya Parishat in Karnataka.

G. Raju, a graduate in agricultural engineering from IIT Kharagpur, went on to do his post-graduation from the Institute of Rural Management, Anand. He has been working in the area of community forestry, with particular focus on the community management of natural resources and the benefits accruing to them. He is currently serving as the Managing Director of a community-owned medicinal plants public limited company, which he helped in initiating.

P. Ram Manohar, who graduated from Ayurveda College, Coimbatore, finished his post-graduation at the ALN Rao Memorial Ayurvedic Medical College, Karnataka. After a stint as Senior Research Fellow at the Foundation for Revitalization of Local Health Traditions (FRHLT), Bangalore, he has gone on to become the General Manager (Clinical Research) of the Arya Vaidya Nilayam, Madurai. He is responsible for initiating PADAM (Program for Archiving and Documenting Ayurvedic Medicine), an Indo-Japanese project that was launched in August 2001 to document the medical traditions of India.

Suma T. S., an Environmental Sciences graduate, completed her post-graduation in Botany at the University of Bangalore. In 1998, she joined the Foundation for Revitalization of Local Health Traditions as part of the project team for Documentation and Rapid Assessment of Local Health Traditions (DALHT). Her professional interests include developing participatory approaches for mainstreaming local health traditions as well as conservation of medicinal plants.

Abbreviations

CAM	–	Complementary and Alternative Medicine
CBD	–	Convention on Biological Diversity
CCRAS	–	Central Council for Research in Ayurveda and Siddha
CCRH	–	Central Council for Research in Homeopathy
CCRNY	–	Central Council for Research in Naturopathy and Yoga
CCRUM	–	Central Council for Research in Unani Medicine)
DLHT	–	Documentation of Local Health Traditions
FRLHT	–	Foundation for Revitalisation of Local Health Traditions
GMP	–	Good Manufacturing Practice
GO	–	Government Organisations
GOI	–	Government of India
ICMR	–	Indian Council for Medical research
IPR	–	Intellectual Property Rights
ISM	–	Indian Systems of Medicine
IT	–	Information Technology
ITA	–	Information Transfer Agreement
KHG	–	Kitchen Herbal Garden
LHT	–	Local Health Traditions
MPCP	–	Medicinal Plant Conservation Parks
MTA	–	Material Transfer Agreement
NGO	–	Non-government organisations
PRA	–	Participatory Rural Appraisal
RALHT	–	Rapid Assessment of Local Health Traditions
SHG	–	Self Help Group
TBA	–	Traditional Birth Attendant
TBS	–	Traditional Bonesetter
TSM	–	Traditional Systems of Medicine
VRP	–	Village Resource Person

Glossary

Ācaraṇa	Practice
Acetana	Consensus
Acintīta	Un-thought
Acintya	Beyond thought
Adhiti	Memorising
Agadatantra	Branch dealing with poisons
Agni	Fire — one of the five existential principles
Agni karma	Cauterisation
Āhāra	Food
Āhāropaśaya	Confirming diagnosis through response to food
Ākāśa	Space — one of the five existential principles
Ākṛti	Shape
Alpadoṣa	With less *dosa*
Āma	Undigested material
Ambatta	A community in south India
Ambattaiyār	A community in south India
Amla	Sour
Amlaseva	Consuming sour food
Amlodgāra	Sour belching
Anala	Fire
Aṅgulī	Finger (a unit of measurement)
Añjana	Application for the eye
Anumāna	Inference
Ānūpa	Wetland

Ap	Water — one of the five existential principles
Apasmāra	Epileptic conditions
Apathya	Unwholesome
Āpta	Seer or highly knowledgeable person
Aptopadesa	Statement of authority in a branch of knowledge
Arśa	Haemorrhoids
Aruci	Loss of appetite
Asthi	Bone tissue
Asthisandhanākṛt	Healing bone fractures
Ātapa	Exposure to ṣunrays
Atisāra	Diarrhoea
Auḍbhida	Plants
Ausadha	Drug
Auṣadha nirmāṇa	Production of medicine
Ausadhī sūkta	Rig Vedic hymn on medicinal plants
Avasthā	Stage
Avega avasthā	A disease stage
Avipāka	Indigestion
Avyakta	That which is not manifest - in Samkhya philosophy
Āyusya	Good for longevity of life
Bahudoṣa	With profuse *dosa*
Bala	Strength
Bāla cikitsā	Paediatrics
Bālagraha	Afflictions of children
Baletodhisuvudu	A custom in south India
Bālya	Toner

Balya	Childhood
Bhagnasandhāna	Healing fractures
Bhaisajya kalpanā	Science of pharmacy
Bhakṣaṇam	Food/intake
Bhasma	Baked powder
Bhautika	Pertaining to five elements
Bheda	Disruption and complication phase
Bhedana	Breaking
Bodhaka	Revealing
Bodham	Contemplation
Brahma	God of creation
Bṛṃhaṇa	Nourishing body tissues
Caladoṣa	*Dosa* which is mobile
Caya	Accumulative phase
Cchedana	Cutting
Cetana	Consciousness
Chakkiliar	A community in south India
Chuzhali	Non-specific fits
Dāha	Burning sensation
Daivavyapāsraya	Spiritual therapy
Daṃṣtra cikitsā	Toxicology
Danta cikitsā	Treatment of teeth
Deśa	Habitat
Deśa sātmya	Habituated by place
Deśa vikalpa	Differential knowledge of habitat
Deśyokti	Regional usage

Dhānya	Grains
Dhārā	Continuous pouring of oil or any other medicated material either on body or on the head
Dhātu	Body tissue
Dīpana	Improving digestive fire
Divyauṣadhi	Divine herbs
Dondi	One of the surgical instruments used in eye diseases
Doṣa	Three physiological principles in the body
Doṣakarma	Drug action on the *dosa*
Dravya	Substance
Dravya vijñāna	Study of drug substances
Dravyaguna vijñāna	Ayurvedic pharmacology
Dūṣya	Body tissues
Dūtalakṣaṇa	Signs of messenger
Gandha	Smell
Gaurava	Heaviness
Graha cikitsā	Psychiatry (also treating evil afflictions)
Grāhi	Inducing constipation
Gso-rig-pa	Tibetan medicine
Gulma	Tumour-like presentations of body
Guṇa	Quality
Guru	Heavy/teacher
Gutika	Pills
Hakim	Physician
Harita	Vegetable
Hṛddāha	Heartburn

Hṛdroga	Ailment of heart
Hṛdya	Good for heart
Ikṣu	Sugarcane
Ilakkam	Non-specific fits
Indriya	Senses
Jala	Water
Jāṅgala	Dry land with specified features
Jaṅgama	Animal substances
Jarā cikitsā	Rejuvenation
Jātaka śāstram	Astrology
Jatharavraṇa	Ulceration in the stomach
Jātiliṅga	Reproductive characteristics of a plant species
Jīvana	Good for life
Jvara	Types of fevers
Kāla	Time/season
Kālakṛta (bala)	(Strength) acquired by time
Kalpanā	Pharmaceutical preparation
Kāma	Lust
Kannu vaidyar	Eye physician
Kanthadāha	Burning sensation in the throat
Kaṇṭhya	Good for throat
Kapha	One of the three *dosas*
Kaphapittahara	Pacifying body principles — *kapha, pitta*
Karkidaka kanji	A medicated porridge taken in rainy season
Karma	Action
Karma virodha	Incompatibility

Kāsa	Cough
Kaṣāya	Astringent/decoction
Katti	A surgical instruments used for treating eye diseases
Kaṭu	Pungent
Kaumāra	Adolescence
Kāvu	Sacred grove
Kāvya	Poetry
Kāya cikitsa	General medicine
Klama	Lethargy
Kledana	Liquifying
Kopanam	Aggravating
Kṛmi	Worms
Krodha	Anger
Ksanadi	Divisions of time
Ksira	Milk
Kṣut	Hunger
Kulasātmya	Habituated by family
Kuruba	A community in south India
Kuṣṭha	Skin diseases with involvement other tissues
Kuṭīprāveśika	A type of rejuvenation achieved by confining oneself to a specially designed house
Laghu	Light
Laṅghana	Depleting
Lavana	Salt
Līna doṣa	*Dosa* which is latent
Lobha	Greed

Loka svāsthya Paramparā	Local health traditions
Mada	Intoxication
Madhura	Sweet
Majjā	Marrow
Mala	Waste matter
Malamūtraśodhaka	Eliminating waste materials
Māmsa	Muscle tissue/meat
Māmsavardhaka	Increasing *mamsa*
Mānasikaroga	Mental diseases
Manda	Dull
Māruta	Wind
Mātrā	Measurement
Mātsarya	Jealousy
Meda	Adipose tissue
Medhya	Good for intellect
Medohara	Cures fat tissue related disorders
Moha	Delirium/delusion
Mṛgāyurveda	Branch of Ayurveda dealing with treatment of animals
Mṛga vaidya	Veterinary healer
Mūrccha	Loss of consciousness
Mūtra	Urine
Nāḍi	Pulse
Nāma	Name
Nāmamāla	String of names
Nasya	Nasal medication

Netra cikitsa	Ayurvedic ophthalmology
Netrābhiṣyanda	Conjunctivitis
Netraroga	Disease of eye
Netravraṇa	Wound in the eye
Nidāna	Aetiology
Nighantu	Lexicon
Nirāma avasthā	Stage of disease without *ama*
Okasātmya	Habituated by practice
Ottamarunnu	Single drug
Pācaka	Improving digestion
Padārtha	Existential principles which are seven in number
Padārtha vijnanā	Study of existential principles
Pāka	Transformation
Panca rasa	Five tastes
Pancakarma	Fivefold methods of treatment in Ayurveda
Pancamahābhūta	Five elements or formative principles
Pāṇḍu	Anaemic conditions
Paradevatā	Family deity
Paramparā	Lineage
Parayar	A community in south India
Parīkṣa	Examination
Pārthiva	Mineral substances
Pātañjala yoga sūtra	Aphorisms written by the sage Patanjali on yoga sastra
Pathya	Wholesome
Pettichi	Midwife
Phalam	Effect/fruit

Pīḍana	Crushing
Pitta	One of the three *dosas*
Pittakṛt	Aggravating *pitta*
Pittaprakopānna	Pitta aggravating food
Pittaśāmaka	Pacifying pitta
Prabhāva	Special pharmacological action
Pracāraṇa	Promote
Prakopa	Aggravation
Prakṛti	Constitution
Pramana	Measurement
Prameha	Diabetic types
Prasannamana	Equilibrium of mind
Prasannātmā	State of pure awareness
Prasannendriya	Sensory equilibrium
Prasara	Spreading of a pathological condition
Prasūti tantra	Obstetrics
Pratikriyā	Antidote
Prayoga	Application
Prīṇana	Pleasing
Pṛithivi	Earth — one of the five existential principles
Rāhukāla	Specific time of the day according to astrology
Rājasika	Psychological constitution
Rakta	Blood
Raktadoṣahara	Pacifying blood tissue disorders
Raktamokṣa	Bloodletting
Raktapitta	Disorders of blood, bleeding disorders

Raktaprasādana	Nourishing blood tissue
Raktārśa	Bleeding piles
Rasa	Taste (also first body tissue)
Rasaśāstra	Branch of Ayurveda dealing with mercury, sulphur, etc.
Rasāyana	Rejuvenative
Roga	Disease
Roga vijñāna	Pathology
Rogaghnata	Effect on disease
Ropaṇa	Healing
Rucya	Improving taste
Rūdhi	Customary usage
Rūkṣa	Rough
Rūpa	Form/full blown symptoms of a disease
Sacetana	Living
Sādhāraṇa	Ordinary land
Sadravya cikitsā	Treatment with drugs
Sahaja (bala)	Natural (strength)
Śāka	Vegetable
Salākā	An instrument
Salya cikitsā	Surgical treatment
Sāma	Equilibrium
Sama avasthā	Disease stage with *ama*
Samadhātu	Equilibrium of body tissues
Samadoṣa	Equilibrium of three *dosa*
Samagni	Equilibrium of metabolic functions

Samamalakriyā	Equilibrium of eliminative system
Śamana	Pacifying
Sāmañya	Generality
Samavāya	Inherence, inseparable connection
Saṁgraha	Compendium
Saṁgrahaṇa vidhi	Rules for collection of drugs
Saṁgrāhī	Constipative
Saṁhita	Treatise
Samkhya	A school of Indian philosophy
Saṁpradāya	Tradition
Saṁprāpti	Complete manifestation of a disease
Samūham	Society
Sañatana	Unchanging
Sankranti habba	Harvest festival in Karnataka
Santarpaka	Nourishing
Sapta	Seven
Śāra	Fluid in nature
Śarira	Anatomy
Śāstra	Surgical instrument
Śāstra	Indian sciences
Sātmya	Habituated
Sattvāvajaya	Psychological treatment
S̄attvika	Psychological constitution
Siddhānta	Principle
Siddhar	Physician in Siddha medicine
Śiṣya	Disciple

Śīta	Cold
Sneha	Love
Snehana	Oleation
Snehapana	Intake of oils/unctuous materials as part of the treatment
Snigdha	Unctuous
Śodhana	Eliminating
Śopha	Oedema
Śoṣaṇa	Drying
Śothahara	Anti-oedema
Sramsana	Laxative
Stambhana	Blocking
Stanyaśodhana	Purifying breast milk
Sthānasaṁsraya	Localisation phase of a disease
Śukra	Reproductive tissue/semen
Śukrala	Increasing semen
Śūla	Abdominal colic
Svarasa	Juice
Śvāsa	Breathing disorders
Svasthavṛtta	Preventive medicine in Ayurveda
Svāsthya	To be established in oneself, natural state
Sveda	Sweat
Svedana	Fomentation
Taila	Oil
Tamakaśvāsa	Asthma
Tamasika	A type of psychological constitution
Tapasvi	Hermitage

Tarka	System or doctrine on reasoning
Tattva	Principle
Tīkṣṇa	Sharp
Tikta	Bitter
Tiktāmlodgāra	Bitter and sour belching
Tridoṣa	Three physiological principles of the body
Tridoṣahara	Pacifying all three principles
Tṛṣṇanivaraṇa	Quenching thirst
Tṛt	Thirst
Tvacya	Good for the skin tissue
Unmada	Mental disorders
Upadeśa	Advice
Upamāna	Comparative logic
Upaśaya	Therapeutic response of diagnostic value
Upaśoṣaṇa	Depleting, drying
Uppara	A community in south India
Ūrdhvāṅga cikitsā	Treatment for ear, nose, throat and eye (disorders above the shoulder region)
Ūrjaskara	Strengthening
Uṣṇa	Heat
Utkleśa	A stage in manifestation of disease
Utpattisthāna	Place of origin
Vaidya	Physician
Vaiśeṣika	A school of Indian philosophy
Vājīkaraṇa	To increase sexual potency
Valakāppu	A custom in south India

Vamana	Vomiting
Vaṇṇān	A community in south India
Vārdhakya	Old age
Vargīkaraṇa	Classification
Varmakalai	Knowledge of *varma* (*marma* — vital points) in the body
Varṇa	Colour
Varti	Wick/pill
Vasanta ṛtu	Spring season
Vāsti	Enema
Vata	One of the three *dosas*
Vatarakta	Arthritic conditions
Vatatapika	A type of *rasayana* without much restrictions
Vaya	Age
Vāyu	Air — one of the five existential principles
Vega avasthā	A disease stage
Vettai	White discharge
Vidāhyanna	Food causing burning sensation
Vikṛti	Imbalance/disorder
Vināyaka puja	Offering to Lord Ganesa
Vireka	Purgation
Viruddhānna	Incompatible food
Vīrya	Potency or power of action
Viṣa	Poison
Viṣama	Irregular
Visarpa	Skin diseases, scabies

Viṣavaidya	Poison healer
Viśeṣa	Specificity
Vṛkṣāyurveda	Branch of Ayurveda dealing with plant treatment
Vṛṣya	Aphrodisiac
Vyādhihara	Curing the disease
Vyādhyavasthā	Stages of disease
Vyākhyā	Critical commentary
Vyakta	Manifest world in Samkhya philosophy
Vyakti	Manifestation phase of a disease
Vyavahāra	Practice
Vyavahārāyurveda	Medical jurisprudence
Vyāyāma	Exercise
Yauvana	Youth
Yoga	Formulation / a school of Indian philosophy
Yoga śāstra	A school of Indian philosophy
Yukti	Application
Yuktikṛta (bala)	(Strength) acquired by systematic routine
Yuktivyapāśraya	Treatment with drugs

Appendix

Charts on Materia Medica

The Indian systems of medicine (both folk and codified) use about 8,000 medicinal plants. The maximum number is used by the folk tradition, followed by Ayurveda, Siddha, Unani, Homeopathy, Tibetan and Modern respectively (see Table 1).

1 Medicinal Plants in Indian Traditional Medicine

	Ayurveda	Folk	Homeopathy	Modern	Siddha	Tibetan	Unani
Ayurveda	1769	731	164	55	743	271	653
Folk	731	4671	147	56	635	201	486
Homeopathy	164	147	482	60	142	70	155
Modern	55	56	60	105	41	17	50
Siddha	743	635	142	41	1121	227	486
Tibetan	271	201	70	17	227	279	227
Unani	653	486	155	50	486	224	751

Source: FRLHT database.

2 List of Animals Mentioned in Ayurvedic Literature

Sanskrit name	English name	Zoological name
Aja	Goat	*Capra hircus*
Ambukukkuti	Moor Hen	*Gullinula chloropus*
Anadvan	Bull	*Bos taurus*
Angaracudaka		
Ankapada	Bat	Order: *Chiroptera*

Sanskrit name	English name	Zoological name
Ara	Avocet	*Recurvirostra avocetta*
Asva	Horse	*Equas caballus*
Asvatara	Mule	
Atyuha		
Avakara		
Avi	Sheep	*Ovis aries*
Babhru	Brown mongoose	*Herpestes fuscus*
Balaka	Crane	*Grus grus*
Bhasa	Breaded Vulture	
Bheka	Frog	
Bhramara	Bee	*Apis* sp.
Bhrngaraja	Shrike (rufous backed)	*Lanius schach*
Cakora	Crow pheasant	*Centropus sinensis*
Cakravaka	Ruddy sheldrake	*Tadorna ferrugenea*
Camara	Yak	*Bos grunniens*
Caruska		
Casa	Indian roller	*Coracias benghalensis*
Cataka	Tree sparrow	
Catuspada	Quadrupeds	
Cillata	Water shrew	
Cirati	Babbler	*Turdoides* sp.
Culuki	Gangetic dolphin	*Platanisia gangetica*
Damstrin		
Dhumika	Owlet	*Athene brama*
Dindimanaka	Toucan	

Sanskrit name	English name	Zoological name
Dundubhi	Grey hornbill	*Tokus birostris*
Dvikakuda	Two-humped camel	
Dvipin	Panther	*Panthera pardus*
Ena	Fawn deer	
Gandupada	Earthworm	
Gaudheyaka	Lizard	
Gavaya	Gayal	
Ghandaka		
Girivartaka	Hill quail	*Ophrysia supercilosa*
Go	Cow	*Bos taurus*
Godha	Iguana	
Gokarna	Cow-eared deer	
Gonarda	Hill partridge	
Gopaputra	Cow-bird	
Grdhra	Vulture	*Gyps bengalensis*
Grhagodha	House lizard	*Hemidactylus* sp.
Hamsa	Swan	*Cygnus* sp.
Haridraka		
Harina	Black buck	*Antelope cervicarpa*
Hastin	Elephant	*Elephas maximus*
Indrabha	Hedge sparrow	*Passer* sp.
Indragopa	Red insect	*Mutella occidentalis*
Jahaka		
Jalauka	Leech	*Hirundo medicinalis*

Sanskrit name	English name	Zoological name
Jambuka	Jackal	*Canis aureus*
Jarjara		
Jati		
Jivajivaka	Peacock pheasant	*Pavo cristatus*
Kadali	Marmot	*Marmota* sp.
Kadamba	Grey-leg goose	*Anas anas/anser anser*
Kairata		
Kaka	Crow	*Corvus* sp.
Kakamadgu		
Kakatundaka	River tern	*Sterna aurantia*
Kakulimrga	Python	*Python molurus*
Kalapucchaka	Black-tailed deer	
Kalavinka	Sparrow	*Passer* sp.
Kamakali	Tropic bird	
Kanabha		
Kanakapota		
Kanku		
Kapardika		*Cyprea moneta*
Kapinjala	Grey partridge	*Francolinus pondicerianus*
Kapota	Pigeon	*Columba livia*
Karandava	White-fronted goose	*Anser albifrons*
Karkataka		*Seilla serrata*
Kartkataka	Crab	
Kasturi	Musk	*Moschus*

Sanskrit name	English name	Zoological name
Katumatsya		
Kesarin	Curlew	*Burhinus oedicnemus*
Khanga	Rhinoceros	*Rhinoceros unicornis*
Khara	Ass	*Equus hemionus*
Kharavrsabha	Jackass	
Kokila	Koel	*Eudynamis scolopacea*
Kottakaraka	Barking deer	*Muntiacus muntjak*
Koyasti	Pond heron – paddy bird	*Ardeola grayii*
Krakara	Snipe	*Gallinago* sp.
Kraunca	Demoiselle crane	*Anthropoides virgo*
Krkalasa	Lizard	
Krsna Sarpa	Black cobra	*Naja naja*
Ksudra sukti	Oyster	*Crassostrea madrasensis*
Kudyakitaka		
Kukkubha	Crow pheasant	*Centropus sinensis*
Kukkuta	Hen	*Gallus* sp.
Kulinga	Sparrow	*Passer* sp.
Kumbhira	Crocodile	*Crocodylus palustris*
Kuranga	Indian antelope	*Antelope cervicarpa*
Kurara	Fish eagle	*Haliaeetus leucoryphus*
Kurcika	Hedgehog	*Hemiechinus* sp.
Kurma	Tortoise	*Gedchelone* sp.
Laksa	Lac	*Laecifer lacca*
Latusaka	Paradise flycatcher	*Terpsiphone paradisi*
Latva	Pied flycatcher	

Sanskrit name	English name	Zoological name
Lava	Common quail	*Coturnix coturnix*
Lohaprstha	Kingfisher	
Lopaka	Fox	*Vulpes bengalensis*
Luta	Spider	
Madgu	Small cormorant	*Phalacrocorax niger*
Madhuha	Haney buzzard	*Pernis ptilorhyncus*
Mahisa	Buffalo	*Bubalus bubalis*
Makara	Great Indian crocodile (Estuarine)	*Crocodylus porosus*
Maksika	House fly	*Musca domestica*
Manitundaka	Oyster-catcher	*Haemotopus ostrilegus*
Marjara	Cat	*Felis* sp.
Masaka	Mosquito	Family : Culicidae
Matsya	Fish	
Matsyaka	Small fish	
Matta Kokila		
Mayura	Peacock	*Pavo cristatus*
Megharava	Trumpeter swan	Cygrus sp.
Mrgamatrka		
Mrnalakantha	Snake-bird	*Anhinga rufa*
Mukta	Pearl	
Mukta sukti	Oyster	*Pinctada vulgaris*
Musaka	Mouse	*Mus musculis*
Nakha		*Achatina fulica*
Nakula	Mongoose	*Herpestes edwardsi*

Sanskrit name	English name	Zoological name
Nandimukha	Flamingo	*Phoenicopterus roseus*
Nemi		
Nyanku	Hog deer	*Axis porcinus*
Pakahamsa	Mute swan	
Pakkara	Green barbet	*Megalamia zeylanica*
Paksin	Bird	
Pandavika	Wood pigeon	*Columba punicea*
Parvata	Dove	
Pasu	Beast	
Patanga	Flying insect	
Pipilika	Ant	
Plava	Pelican	*Pelicanus* sp.
Pravala	Coral	*Corallium rubrum*
Priyatmaja	Indian babbler	
Priyavadi		
Prsata	Spotted deer	*Axis axis*
Pundarika		
Pundarikaksa	White-eyed pochard	*Aythya nyroca*
Puskarahva	Lily trotter	
Rajahamsa	Bar headed goose	*Anser indicus*
Raktasirsaka	Purple heron	*Ardea pupusea*
Raktavartmaka	Red jungle fowl	*Gallus gallus*
Rama		*Cervus elaphus*
Rksa	Bear	*Ursa* sp.

Sanskrit name	**English name**	**Zoological name**
Rohini	Common teal	
Rsya		
Ruru	Swamp deer	*Cervus duvauceli*
Sahacarin	Petrel	
Salabha		
Sallaka	Porcupine	*Mystrix indica*
Sambara	Sambar	*Cervus uniclor*
Sambuka	Snail	
Samkha	Conch shell	*Turbinella pyrum*
Samkhanabhi		
Samudraphena	Cuttlefish	
Sankha	Conch	*Turbinella pyrum*
Saphari	A type of fish	
Sarabha	Wapiti	
Saranga	Rose-ringed parakeet	*Psittucula krameri*
Sarapada	Stork	
Sarari	Skimmer bird	*Rhyncops albicollis*
Sarasa	Indian crane	*Grus grus*
Sarika	Mynah	*Acridotheres tristis*
Sarpa	Snake	
Sasa	Rabbit	*Lepus* sp.
Sasaghni	Golden eagle	
Satapatra	Black woodpecker	*Dryocopus javensis*
Siddhartha		

Sanskrit name	English name	Zoological name
Simha	Lion	*Panthera leo*
Sisumara	Estuarine crocodile	*Crocodyus porosus*
Srmara	Wild bear	*Ursa* sp.
Sthulanakula		
Suka	Parakeet	*Psittacula* sp.
Sukti	Pearl oyster	
Sumukha		
Svadamstra	Mouse deer	*Tragulus meminna*
Svavid	Pangolin	*Manis crassicaudata*
Syena	Hawk	*Accipter* sp.
Taila maksika	Telini fly	*Mylabris chicorii*
Taraksu	Heyna	*Hyaena hyaena*
Timingila	Whale	*Balaenoptera musculus*
Tittiri	Red-wattled Lapwing	*Vanellus indicus*
Udra	Catfish	
Uluka	Owl	
Upacakra	Smaller Greek pheasant	
Urana	Wild sheep	*Ovis ammon*
Ustra	Camel	*Camelus aromedarius*
Utkrora	Mallard	*Anas platyrhynchos*
Vaka	Common crane	*Grus grus*
Vanara	Monkey	
Vantada	Dog	*Canis familiaris*
Varada		
Varaha	Hog	

Sanskrit name	English name	Zoological name
Varapota	Small antelope	
Varataka	Cowrie	
Varmin		
Vartaka	Male bustard	*Choriotis nigriceps*
Vartika	Female bustard	
Varttiraka	Rain quail	*Coturnix coromandelica*
Vastra-Krimi	Clothes insects	
Vataha		
Vati	Little grebe	*Tachybaptus ruficollis*
Visvambhara		
Vriscika	Scorpion	
Vrka	Wolf	*Canis lupus*
Vyaghra	Tiger	*Panthera tigris*
Yastika	Sunbird	*Nectariania* sp.
Yuka	Lice	*Pediculus humanus*

3 Minerals and Metals Used in Ayurveda

Group	Name of the material	Types available	Type preferred from natural sources	Historical period	Usages
Group 1	Rasa/ parad (Mercury)	5	Extracted from native cinnabar ore (Hingula)	Samhita period. Used from 500 AD onwards.	Rejuvenation therapy, asthma, cholitis
Group 2	Abhrak (Mica)	16	Krishna vajrabharak	Samhita period. Used from 7th century AD onwards.	Rejuvenation, psychological disorders.
Group 2	Makshik (Copper, pyrite)	3	Swarnmakshik	Sushruta period 100 BC.	Virility, rejuvenation, eye and bladder, heart disorders, prameha, pandoo, shopha.
Group 2	Vimal (Pyrite iron)	3	Kansyavimal	5th century AD Samhita period.	Cures haemorrhoids (internal), liver diseases
Group 4	Gauri-pashan (Arsenic dioxide)	2/3	Spatikabha	Rasashastra period, 5th to 16th AD.	Typhoid, rhumatoid arthritis, venereal diseases, mahakushtha.

Group	Name of the material	Types available	Type preferred from natural sources	Historical period	Usages
Group 5	Suvarna (Gold)	12	Khanija	Known since Vedic time. Used to an extent from Samhita period. Used in many formulations during Rasa era.	Rejuvenation, detoxifier, virility, enhances brain capacity, anti-aging.
Group 5	Loha (Iron)	3	Kanthloha	Pre-Vedic period – post Vedic period	Liverdisorder, anti-aging, prameha, raktavaha srotas.
Group 6	Mandoor (Iron oxide)	3	Hundred years old ore	Known and used since Samhita period	Paediatric drug, for pandoo, kamala, shotha (Hepatitis of all types).
Group 7	Shankha (Conch shell)	2	Seashell – dakshinavarta	Known and used since Samhita period.	Grahani (colitis), pimple and acne, cataract and glaucoma.

Group	Name of the material	Types available	Type preferred from natural sources	Historical period	Usages
Group 7	Mukta (Pearl)	8	Seashell pearl	Known and used religiously since Vedic period. Used during Samhita period	Detoxifying and soothing drug, balya, rejuvenation.
Group 8	Manikya (Ruby)	2	Padmarag	Used since Vedic era from astrological viewpoint as ornament; used as medicine since Caraka samhita.	Rejuvenation, virility, brain tonic and cardio tonic.
Group 9	Suryakanth (Sunstone)			Known and used after 10th century AD	Works on CNS, rasayan, kapha vatagraha.

4 Animals in Siddha Medicine

1 Attai (leech)

2 Akaleli or valaiyeli (moderat—Nesokia indica)

3 Alkattippatci (red-wattled lapwing, sandpiper)

4 Amai (tortoise)

5 Ampar (pigeons reared in houses

6 Antamanpanr (Andaman pig)

7 Antankakkai (Indian raven, carrion crow)

8 Arakku (lac)

9 Arru min (river fish)

10 Arupatankoli (a hen which lays eggs every 2 months)

11 Ayirai (herring)

12 Campankoli (a species of fowl)

13 Canna kuni (common shrimp: small prawn)

14 Cannakkentai (small carp of stunted growth)

15 Cavvatu (civet)

16 Cel kentia (shell carp)

17 Cemmai nira matar mulaippal

18 Cemmai nira pacumpal

19 Cemmariyattu iraicci (sheep)

20 Cennay (red dog)

21 Cevarkoli (cock)

22 Cevveli (antelope rat)

23 Cimai nay (European dog)

24 Cimai onay (European wolf)

25 Cimaippanri (German boar)

26 Cinappanri (chine hog)

27 Cirraral (sand eel)

28 Cirupuli iraicci

29 Cittukkuruvi (small sparrow)

30 Civippatci

31 Coki

32 Cura karuvatu (dried shark)

33 Curaippatci (a kind of bird)

34 Curumpu (milk fish)

35 Eli iraicci (rat)

36 Elumpu (bone)

37 Eri min (lake fish)

38 Erumaippal (buffalo milk)

39 Intira kopa pucci (lady's fly- scarlet moth)

40 Iraippeli (a kind of rat whose bite causes sharpness of breath)

41 Iral (shrimp)

42 Irappacuvin pal

43 Kaccar karuvatu (fish salted and dried)

44 Kakkai ney

45 Kalaiman iraicci (antelope)

46 Kalleli (rufescent tree rat)

47 Kalutaippal (donkey milk)

48 Kanankoli (small jungle fowl)

49 Kapilai nira pacumpal

50 Kapilaveli (Mus brunneus found in houses, godowns, etc)

51 Karampacumpal

52 Karati iraicci (bear)

53 Kareli (black rat)

54 Karralai min (a sea fish, Jew – fish – Sciaena genus)

55 Karu vauval (black flat sea fish – this is not good for health)

56 Karumai nira matar mulaippal

57 Karumai nira pacumpal

58 Karunkokku (a stork with a black bill)

59 Karunkoli (a fowl whose skin and bones are black)

60 Karunkuruvi (black sparrow)

61 Kasturi (musk)

62 Katai (quail)

63 Katal iranci

64 Katal kelirru

65 Katal nantu (sea crab)

66 Katalnay (sea dog)

67 Kataman iraicci (wild cow)

68 Katarpanri (sea hog)—a type of fish

69 Kattatu (forest goat)

70 Katteli (jungle rat)

71 Kattu koli (jungle fowl)

72 Kattunay (wild dog)

73 Kattuppanri iraicci (boar)

74 Kavutari (Indian partridge)

75 Kentai (carp)

76 Kilankan min (Indian whiting)

77 Kileli (jerbora rat)

78 Kiluvai (common teal)

79 Kinarru min (well fish)

80 Kiri iraicci (mongoose)

81 Kiruttippatci (a kind of bird)

82 Kocu ullan (small snipe)

83 Kokku (crane)

84 Koli (domestic hen)

85 Kollik karuvatu (dried and salted Indian turbot)

86 Komacaiyum pacumpal

87 Kompai (poligar dog)

88 Komputten

89 Konay (Indian wolf)

90 Korai ullan (a species of long snipe)

91 Korocanai (bezoar)

92 Kotiyattu iraicci (a species of long-legged goat)

93 Kottan (rock horned owl)

94 Kulaikkata (a kind of stork with a short or no tail)

95 Kulam min (pond fish)

96 Kuravai

97 Kurumbattu iraicci (a short, woolly sheep with crumpled horns)

98 Kutiraippal (horse milk)

99 Kuyil (koel)

100 Malaitten (honey from the mountains)

101 Malaiyatu (mountain goat)

102 Man iraicci (deer)

103 Manaippura (pigeons reared in houses)

104 Manaitten (honey extracted from beehives formed within homes)

105 Manippura (a variety of dove)

106 Maranay iraicci (a species of dog living on trees)

107 Marappontutten

108 Maraveli (tree rat)

109 Mataiyan (a water bird, Ardea)

110 Matappura (domestic pigeon)

111 Matavai (grey mullet)

112 Matu iraicci (cattle)

113 Matu min (fish from deep parts of a river)

114 Mayari min

115 Mayil (peacock)

116 Meluku (wax)

117 Miruka kompu (horn)

118 Motteli (Mus alexandrinus found in roofs of houses and on tops of buildings)

119 Mucal iraicci (rabbit)

120 Mucuru muttai (the egg of a red ant which has its nest in trees. The one on the tree of bassia longifolia is considered best for medicinal use)

121 Mulaippal vennai (butter from breast milk)

122 Mullampanri iraicci (porcupine)

123 Mulleli (bristle rat or hedgehog)

124 Munram yirru pacumpal

125 Mutalai iraicci (crocodile)

126 Mutpanri (Bengal porcupine)

127 Muttuccippi (oyster shell)

128 Namittuppatci (a kind of unknown bird used in convalescence and for treating tuberculosis)

129 Nankamirru pacumpal

130 Narai (heron)

131 Naraiman kapilai pacumpal

132 Narinay (fox)

133 Nattai (snail)

134 Nattu nay (country dog)

135 Nattupanri (country pig)

136 Neruppukkoli (ostrich)

137 Neyttoli (small fish containing much fat, therefore not easily digestible)

138 Nirkkakkai (crow of the pelican family)

139 Nirkkoli (waterfowl)

140 Nirnay (water dog)

141 Olai vali karuvatu (a silvery cuttlefish)

142 Onan ney

143 Onay (wolf)

144 Ottai mor (camel buttermilk)

145 Paccaippura (green pigeon – Crocopus chlorigaster)

146 Pacu ney (cow ghee)

147 Pakarpacuvinpal

148 Pal (milk)

149 Palakarai (marine shell)

150 Pallaiyattu iraicci (an undersized goat)

151 Pallattu ney

152 Panri ney (boar ghee)

153 Paranay (pariah dog)

154 Parattaiyar mulaippal

155 Peraral (a kind of fish)

156 Peruccali iraicci (bandicoot)

157 Pettai koli (hen fowl)

158 Pinkan

159 Ponnantattan (a bird whose flesh is edible. It cures skin diseases, venereal diseases and internal heat)

160 Puli iraicci (tiger)

161 Punai iraicci (cat)

162 Punakam (earthworm)

163 Punuku cattam (the ventricle of the civet cat where the perfume is generated)

164 Purrutten (honey from the anthill)

165 Putareli (bush rat)

166 Taippal (mother's milk)

167 Tara (a kind of duck, teal)

168 Tavittuppura (bran dove)

169 Tirukkai (a kind of large sea fish; Trygon genus)

170 Tukkunankuruvi (Indian tailorbird)

171 Tunkeli (rat, whose bite induces sleep)

172 Ullamin (sable fish)

173 Ullan (common snipe)

174 Uluvai (mud fish)

175 Urkkuruvi (village sparrow)

176 Urppanri iraicci (village pig)

177 Utumpu iraicci (water lizard)

178 Valai (a fish; wallago uttu)

179 Vanampati (Indian skylark)

180 Vankoli (turkey)

181 Vannappura

182 Varaiyattu iraicci

183 Varappeli (ridge rat)

184 Varippura (a kind of dove)

185 Vattu (goose)

186 Vayal nantu (field crab)

187 Vayaleli (field rat)

188 Vellai canku (white conch)

189 Vellai vauval (white flat sea-fish)

190 Vellattu mutiram (goat urine)

191 Velleli iraicci (grey rat)

192 Venmai nira pacumpal

193 Vennai (butter)

194 Venpura (white dove used in the treatment of leucoderma, eczema etc.

195 Vettainay (hound)

196 Vicculi (a small swift bird)

197 Vilanku min (eel)

198 Vinkeli (a rat whose bite causes swelling)

199 Viral min (a fresh water fish – murrel – ophicephalus striatus)

200 Vitteli (house rat)

201 Yanai muttiram (elephant urine)

5 Metals and Minerals in Siddha Medicine

The *siddhars* talk about 220 metal and mineral drugs that they group under the following categories:

Ulokam —11 (metals)

Patanam — 64 (poisonous compounds)

Karacaram — 25 (salts and alkalis)

Uparasam — 120 (natural substances)

Ulokam — 11

Iyarkai ulokam (naturally available metals)

1 Cempu (copper)	4 Nakam (zinc)	7 Velli (silver)
2 Irumpu (iron)	5 Tankam (gold)	8 Velliyam (tin)
3 Kariyam (lead)	6 Urukku (steel)	

Ceyarkkai ulokam (prepared metals)

1 Pittalai (brass)	2 Tara (mixture of Copper and Lead)	3 Venkalam (bronze)

Karacaram — 25

Iyarkai uppu (natural salts)

1 Cinam	5 Katalnurai	9 Puniru
2 Cutan	6 Minampar	10 Valayaluppu
3 Kalluppu	7 Paccaik karpuram	
4 Kariyuppu	8 Ponnampar	

Ceyarkkaiuppu (prepared salts)

1 Catticcaram	6 Kacilavanam	11 Pitalavanam
2 Cintulavanam	7 Kaycculavanam	12 Pottiluppu
3 Ekamparaccaram	8 Kentilavanam	13 Tilalavanam
4 Evatcaram	9 Kentiuppu	14 Turucu
5 Intuppu	10 Navaccaram	15 Venkaram

Patanam — 64

Iyarkai patanam

1 Amirtam
2 Ancanam
3 Appirakam
4 Avu pal
5 Calankam
6 Canku
7 Carakantam
8 Cilai
9 Cilamatam
10 Cirapantam
11 Citankam
12 Cuta patanam
13 Ilinkam
14 Kaccalam
15 Kantakam
16 Kantam
17 Karataka patanam
18 Karmukil
19 Karpari
20 Karpatanam
21 Kauri
22 Kolakam
23 Kutiraippal
24 Mirutaram
25 Palntirukam
26 Talakam
27 Talampam
28 Totti
29 Tuttam
30 Vaikirantam
31 Vellai
32 Viram

Ceyarkai patanam

1 Aritara vaippu
2 Catilinkam
3 Cavviram
4 Cepputt totti
5 Cora patanam
6 Cutapatanam
7 Ema cinki
8 Erumainattotti
9 Ilavanam
10 Intira patanam
11 Iracitam
12 Iratta cinki
13 Iratta patanam
14 Kakam
15 Kantakam
16 Karumukil
17 Kolittalai kenti
18 Kota cori
19 Kunkuma patanam
20 Mirutarucinki
21 Naka patanam
22 Nilam
23 Panca patci
24 Pavala purru
25 Portotti
26 Puttottut totti
27 Tailam
28 Ti murukal
29 Turucu
30 Tuttam
31 Vanakkenti
32 Vellai

Uparasam — 120

1 Amai
2 Anaikkompu
3 Annapeti
4 Appirakam
5 Astipeti
6 Attukkompu
7 Ayaccilaikkal
8 Calikkiramam
9 Cattirapeti
10 Cemman
11 Cempu malai
12 Cempu man

13 Cenkal
14 Cevvattai
15 Cilavankam
16 Cittakkal
17 Connapeti
18 Cukkan
19 Cukkan kal
20 Cutalaikkal
21 Cutta manal
22 Elimul
23 Elumpu
24 Emaccilai
25 Emaman
26 Erumpu
27 Intirakopam
28 Iracavarttakkal
29 Iracita cilai
30 Irakkal
31 Iya manal
32 Iyaccilai
33 Kakacilai
34 Kalaikkompu
35 Kalmatam
36 Kalnar
37 Kalutai vantu
38 Kantakkal
39 Kantam
40 Kantamiruka kompu
41 Karati
42 Karcuvatu
43 Karppuracccilai
44 Karumanal
45 Karunkal
46 Karutakkal
47 Karuvantu
48 Katalnurai
49 Katarpaci
50 Katturi
51 Kavikkal
52 Kentacilai
53 Kilincal
54 Kolikkal
55 Kometakam
56 Kulavikkuttu man
57 Kuruntakkal
58 Kuruvantu
59 Makkal
60 Man kompu
61 Mancatkal
62 Manikkam
63 Mankicacilai
64 Mankicapeti
65 Mantalirkkal
66 Mantaraccilai
67 Marakatam
68 Mattukkal
69 Mattullompu
70 Mayil
71 Mayir
72 Min elumpu
73 Minminippucci
74 Mutcanku
75 Muttai
76 Muttu
77 Nakaccattai
78 Nakaccilai
79 Nakamanal
80 Nakapaccai
81 Nakaravantu
82 Nantu
83 Nattai
84 Naykkattam
85 Nilam
86 Nilancanakkal
87 Nuttuccippi
88 Ottin tul
89 Paccai
90 Pal
91 Panrikkompu
92 Panrimul
93 Patikakal
94 Pavalam
95 Perocanai
96 Pittalai malai
97 Ponnimilai
98 Punakam
99 Puraveccam
100 Purrampalam
101 Pusparakam
102 Taramalai
103 Tavalai
104 Tavalakkal
105 Tekkal

106 Ten	111 Uvarman	116 Vankaccilai
107 Timinkalam	112 Vaikirantam	117 Vayiram
108 Tirucu	113 Vaituriyam	118 Vellaikkal
109 Ulokamanal	114 Valappakkal	119 Velli manal
110 Uram	115 Vanka manal	120 Venkalamalai

Index

A

B

C

M

N

V

W

Y

Z